WISDOM
in the
SEASONS

First published in 2025 by
Alicky Gravell, in partnership with Whitefox Publishing Ltd
www.wearewhitefox.com
Copyright © Alicky Gravell, 2025

EU GPSR Authorised Representative
LOGOS EUROPE, 9 rue Nicolas Poussin, 17000, LA ROCHELLE, France
E-mail: Contact@logoseurope.eu

ISBN 978-1-917523-49-3
Also available as an eBook
ISBN 978-1-917523-50-9

Alicky Gravell asserts the moral right to be identified as the author of this work.

All rights reserved. No part of this publication may be reproduced, stored in a retrieval system or transmitted in any form or by any means, electronic, mechanical, photocopying, recording or otherwise, without prior written permission of the author.

While every effort has been made to trace the owners of copyright material reproduced herein, the author would like to apologise for any omissions and will be pleased to incorporate missing acknowledgements in any future editions.

Disclaimer: All the information, techniques, skills and concepts contained within this publication are of the nature of general comment only and are not in any way recommended as individual advice. The intent is to offer a variety of information to provide a wider range of choices now and in the future, recognising that we all have widely diverse circumstances and viewpoints. Should any reader choose to make use of the information herein, this is their decision, and the author and publisher/s do not assume any responsibilities whatsoever under any conditions or circumstances. The author does not take responsibility for the business, financial, personal or other success, results or fulfilment upon the readers' decision to use this information. It is recommended that the reader obtain their own independent advice.

All photographs and illustrations in this book © Georgia Lumley, unless otherwise stated.

Designed and typeset by Karen Lilje
Cover design by Heike Schüssler
Project management by Whitefox Publishing

Finding Harmony
in Mind, Body & Nature

WISDOM in the SEASONS

ALICKY GRAVELL
INTEGRATED MIND AND BODY THERAPIST

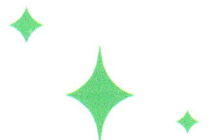

I dedicate this book to those who doubted my capabilities, and told me to quieten down when I had an opinion. You are the reason I am finally showing up, putting words on paper with positive power, better and stronger than ever.

Contents

Preface | ix
Introduction | 1
Important Foundations Before We Begin | 5

Spring | 19
Summer | 45
Autumn | 65
Winter | 89

Now For a Bit of Fun! | 111
Conclusion | 123

Additional Resources | 125
Acknowledgements | 127
About the Author | 129

Preface

I grew up on farms in Leicestershire, Wiltshire and Scotland, but I really wasn't aware of the ever-changing seasons having any effect on me, except the low feeling of going back to school after a long, hot summer. The summer weather always seemed to be hot, didn't it? It's funny, I don't remember cold, rainy days – apart from Scotland at times!

Summer was vegetable-growing time: cutting thistles in the fields to avoid them spreading, alongside long, hazy days of animals, competitions, picnics, swimming in the river and the sea, and sleeping out under the stars. Autumn was spent picking blackberries for jam, apples for stewing and baking. Spring is remembered by smells of freshly mown grass, blossom floating around, daffodils everywhere, and newborn animals joining the motley crew.

In winter, we were outdoors whatever the weather, riding and caring for horses. The days would end earlier and earlier, with less daylight, and we would have hot baths, followed by toast next to the fire. I was fortunate, growing up on a farm, that my mother had the interest and life experience to guide us through childhood whilst abiding to seasonal rhythms. What memories do you have of a particular season?

My mother taught me to live organically and in alignment with the fruits of the Earth, the Moon and the stars. Our nourishment came from nature. She loved sleeping out under the stars, and we all dragged mattresses out on hot summer evenings. My own children love to do this now.

My father was vehemently against pharmaceutical medicines and encouraged natural living. Indeed he was saved from sepsis in the Second World War by champagne of all things! Resveratrol in champagne is said to be anti-inflammatory.

My brother had appalling eczema, so to treat it we had a helping hand from the goats on our farm. The milk and cheese from the goats' milk could make tinctures, prepared by a naturopath, then Chinese herbs and all sorts were added for extra treatment. Goat's milk was perfectly disgusting in my opinion – it is still a joke in my family – but truly effective for eczema. For gut health repair and support, microbes (probiotics) from goat's milk are fabulous for repopulating the gut with good bacteria, building and supporting the gut microbiome, your internal army of defence.

Between 1991 and 1994, I trained and then qualified for a degree equivalent in Traditional Chinese Medicine (TCM) and shiatsu, a form of eastern physio. TCM stems from Asia and is rooted in illness prevention. Using Chinese wisdom and the five-element theory of fire, water, earth, wood and metal can lead to a very simple and balanced life. These three years literally changed my life. I started to view every day through a slightly different lens.

I built on my future career, expanding my skills by qualifying in reflexology, a study and treatment of the body via the feet through reflex zones. By stimulating the feet, one can unblock nerve pathways and help each organ to function properly, healing the body and mind. Shortly after this, I qualified in InterX Therapy for pain and injury healing, then in Emotional Freedom Technique (EFT or tapping), Neuro-Linguistic Programming (NLP) and finally hypnotherapy. Energy healing and reflexology are a powerful integration of body and mind energy techniques. The combination packs a powerful punch! This education and training carried on for the next thirty years and has led me where I am today.

I never imagined I would write a book, but with the encouragement of loyal friends, clients and a supportive family, I decided to be brave and empty my brain onto the page to share my wisdom with you.

PREFACE

This book is packed with easy ideas to balance your energy, enhance your nutrition, nurture your body through each season and improve your knowledge of life. It shows a simple way of living from another perspective, which I have honed through my life. I see many clients in my clinic and people in everyday life who are out of balance, off-centre, confused, and, of course, many who are unwell. There is so much information out there and it is easy to get lost in the detail. We don't need to know everything. You can add a little knowledge for a lot of reward. I promise! I hope you practise well and enjoy. Perhaps this is the start of a journey towards living in harmony with the seasons.

Lots of love, Alicky x

Introduction

'Life is really simple, but we insist on making it complicated.'
Confucius

Most of us live in a state of imbalance. Every day in my work as a therapist of somatic and cognitive healing therapies, I see exhaustion, stress, overwhelm, anxiety, emotional and physical pain, digestion disorders, myalgic encephalomyelitis (M.E.), post-viral fatigue and complications, plus depression, children in distress with tummy ache, bad sleep habits and bullying.

What have we humans done to ourselves?

One easy way to correct our imbalance is to tune into the seasons: living in the ebb and flow of mother nature and the seasons is something we have forgotten. How are you affected by the seasons? It's true that the change of seasons can knock us off balance. We are not designed to work at the same intensity all year round. Our energy will feel different in each season. As the seasons shift, our comfortable routines must change as fresh energy enters the physical body from the natural world. In winter, do you have the feeling of just wanting to climb into bed and wait for spring? I certainly do at times!

Tune into how you feel in each season. Which one suits you best? You may say, 'Oh, summer is the best for everyone.' But this is not so. An example of this comes from when I lived on the equator in East Africa, where there are fewer fluctuations between seasons. Of course, the constant sunshine was joyful, however, I really missed the winter months of holing up next to a fire in the long, dark evenings and taking time to turn inwards, to nourish and reconnect and then re-emerge in spring with joy.

Although we may try, we can't stay static, either mentally or physically. Change is inevitable. Seasons, rhythms, people, issues – life is constantly moving, and learning to ride the ebbs and flows without resistance can be life-changing. When we get stuck, we can be 'searching for that one thing', but we don't know what, or sometimes we just feel 'off'. That's imbalance, take a moment to tune into that thought process and then dive into this book.

There are seasons and rhythms in all parts of our life. This Earth has four unique seasons, leading us from winter to spring through to summer and autumn. Chinese wisdom uniquely believes in five seasons, splitting summer into low summer and high summer. We humans also have seasons throughout our lives, from birth through childhood, to adulthood, and into older age. Spring is the time for creation and growth; summer is full of fruit and abundance; autumn is the contracting season; and winter is the closing.

We see seasons most easily in nature, where the rhythms continue year after year. Nature inspires us, showing us how to blossom and bloom. Living in harmony with the seasons is at the core of Traditional Chinese Medicine (TCM), with devotees basing their life on staying in harmony with nature and the cycles that come with it. Generally, the closer you are to nature, the healthier you become and the more energised and happier you feel.

What you will find in this book

This book guides you through the four main seasons of spring, summer, autumn and winter. I will share with you a seasonal summary of easy and harmonious lifestyle advice from a western and eastern point of view. This knowledge and guidance is drawn from over thirty years of working with patients in my clinic where I practise integrated mind and body energy healing techniques.

INTRODUCTION

In each part of this book, you will find an explanation of each season and the wobbles and disruptions one can feel. The boons and banes as I like to call them are the positives and negatives of the seasons. I don't particularly like using the word negative, so I chose these words to replace them.

Then there is a deeper exploration into our physical human responses to each season. This will be an essential guide for you when looking at the emotional element of the seasons, which is accompanied by an overview of food to incorporate into your meals over the year.

Eastern culture is rooted in illness prevention, but western culture is not. My wish is to bridge the two approaches. I invite you to join me on this adventure and gather fun and simple ideas for living healthy happy days throughout each season.

Nature is a powerful socket to plug into. It is free and all yours to share. Please be curious when you dive in and explore. Have fun with it! Louise Hay, a prolific motivational speaker, wrote 'Take on an idea from the book and use it!' Keep it simple. Simple is profound. By the way, reader, you may disagree with what I write about! Just take what you need from this book.

Important Foundations Before We Begin

There are seasons and rhythms throughout our daily lives. This is a book for working with the energy of the seasons in general. Depending on where you live in the world, your seasons will occur in different months and this will affect the energy around you differently. You will need to take into account your location, the weather, the unique environment and all the other tiny elements that create the energy surrounding you to live your daily life in harmony.

Look around you in each season and see what is abundant in nature. In this fast-paced modern world we have created, we have forgotten the basic function of gathering emotional and physical nourishment during each season. The learning and wisdom to remember is to stay in tune with the energy shifts throughout these sometimes turbulent seasons.

> *'My body is in accord with my mind, my mind with my energies, my energies with my spirit.'*
> LIE YUKOU

Chi or Energy: our life force

Chi or qi can be explained in a few ways; most commonly, we know it as an energy or vital life force that flows through all living things. This energy is metaphysical rather than being directly measurable scientifically. Normal energy from the normal function of your body, your chi, is uniquely yours, but you

WISDOM IN THE SEASONS

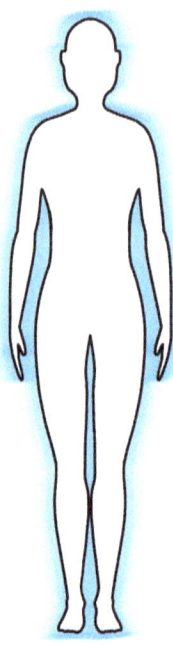

This image shows the chi or energy which surrounds us,
sometimes known as our energy field or aura.

also share it with our planet. We get chi from the ground, Mother Earth, and the universe surrounding us. We breathe it in daily. It flows through us in our blood and meridian channels (or radiant pathways), unseen by the naked eye, energising us throughout the day and night and through the seasons. The state of our physical body and our mind has a big influence on how this energy flows. Traditional Chinese Medicine techniques have been an effective way of healing the body for thousands of years and its focus always starts with the chi. While the chi is the foundation of eastern medical values, western medicine regards the body as just a bag of chemicals and body parts! How little we know – though I do feel there is a tide of change occurring.

As well as guiding you through the seasons, this book will show how we can improve our energy levels, it will guide you to find balance when your energy is too high or low. You may be tired, depressed or have ongoing health issues. You may be hyper-energised and feeling frantic. By nurturing ourselves through the

IMPORTANT FOUNDATIONS BEFORE WE BEGIN

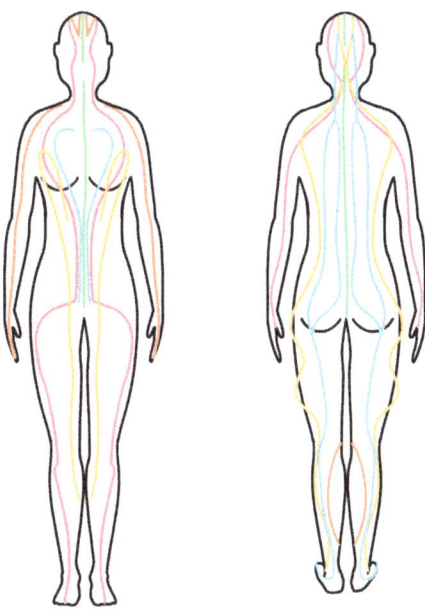

This image shows the map of the energy pathways, called meridians, throughout the body.

seasons, we can improve the smooth flow of chi in and around our bodies to ensure it is moving like a clear stream of water. This balancing of our energy will ensure vigour and love of life.

Chi gung is a form of exercise that will be mentioned throughout this book. It is a combination of movement, mindfulness and breathing to harmonise your vital chi. Daily practice of chi gung will significantly enhance your energy levels by clearing any blockages or stagnation through your meridian system.

Meridians and how they connect through us

Meridian channels or radiant pathways cannot be seen with the naked eye. Energy, or chi, like the blood in arteries, travels along meridians, carrying nourishment and strength. Your chi interconnects all the parts of your body and is essential in maintaining a harmonious balance of energy. The meridians act like motorways for chi energy. They have accurate points along them to stimulate or calm your system. Disease can start when there is a disruption in energy flow or stagnation along these meridians. To open our chi radiant pathways, we must learn the exact points for treatment with acupuncture or shiatsu. With training, the chi can simply be felt by touch.

Some organs are higher up the ranking than others, similar to life really! The heart is the governor. Without your heart, you cannot exist. Whereas, if you lost your spleen, for example, you would not die because your body and energy system would adjust.

Yin and yang

I am sure you have heard these words batted around but might not have really understood what they mean. In eastern philosophy, the energy of yin and yang combined does all the energetic work and excels through cleverness and wisdom. In short, yin and yang are a representation of balance. They complement each other in being opposites and cannot survive without each other: light and heavy, day and night, heat and cold.

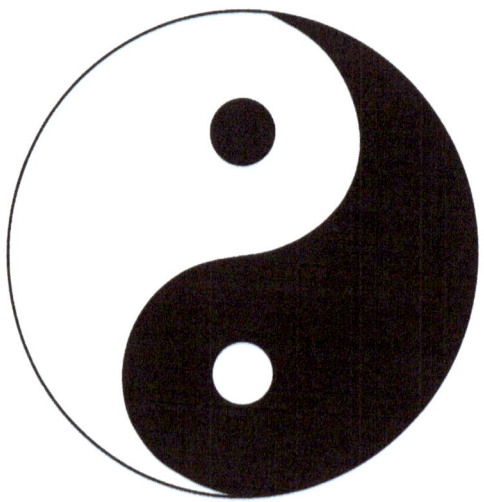

Yin and yang symbol showing the balance of both forces.

IMPORTANT FOUNDATIONS BEFORE WE BEGIN

YIN	YANG
Light	Heavy
Day	Night
Cold	Hot
Soft	Hard
Feminine energy	Masculine energy
Inward	Outgoing
Stillness	Movement

How are our organs are connected to each season?

In Chinese wisdom, the energetic levels of the organs in our body are extremely important. Each organ governs our energy meridians, distributing our chi and connecting all parts of our body to each other. If our veins and arteries are congested, we can feel faint, breathless and weak. The same applies for our chi flow. If we have a blockage in our chi flow, then disease will have a chance to manifest, therefore, it is vital to keep our chi flowing.

This energetic force of chi is in charge of your body's health through the seasons and connects us to nature and our emotional well-being. In simple western terms, we change mood in each season. Happier in the summer, gloomy in the autumn then closing down as we adjust to the colder weather and long dark evenings of winter. Actually, winter can be great and we can adjust to it well. It's the thought of it, really, that incites a low mood. Then there is the anticipation of spring, which has a habit of disappearing as quickly as we glimpse it! Then boom – summer hijacks us with its intensity, we strip off our layers, clear our winter clothes away, and panic it will be over too soon. More often than not

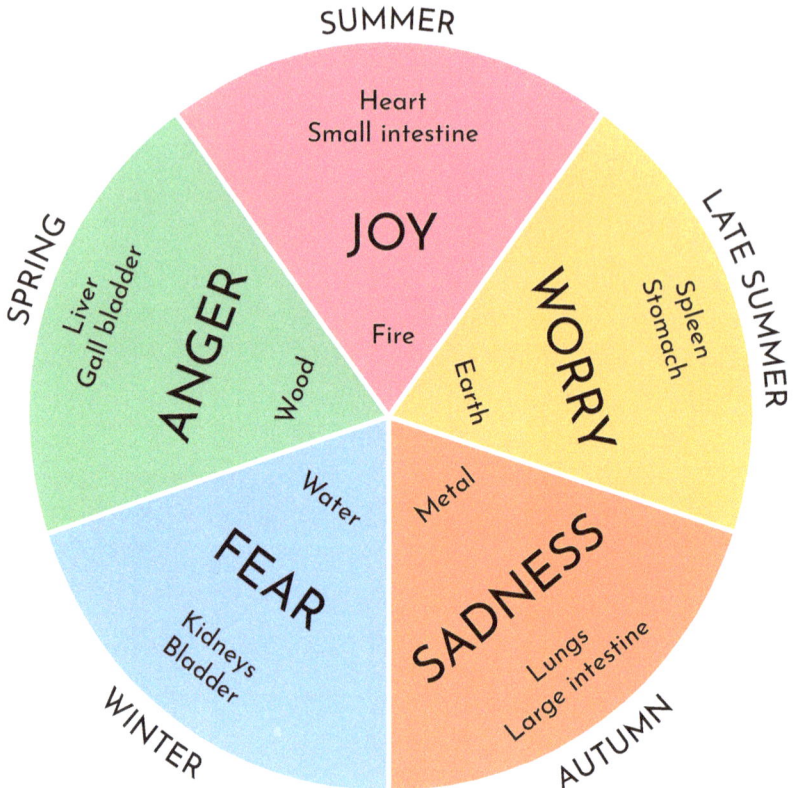

This diagram shows how our organs are connected to each season, along with the element and the main emotion of each season.

there are complaints ... 'Oh, it's too hot, humid, too many bugs and flies!' We never seem to be happy in any season and rarely are we balanced in our feelings. Do you notice that?

Have a think about how you feel in the different seasons. What's your favourite season? Perhaps you love them all and are truly balanced in life. This is rare, normally we dislike a season. Knowing what you feel about each season can help you diagnose your imbalance.

IMPORTANT FOUNDATIONS BEFORE WE BEGIN

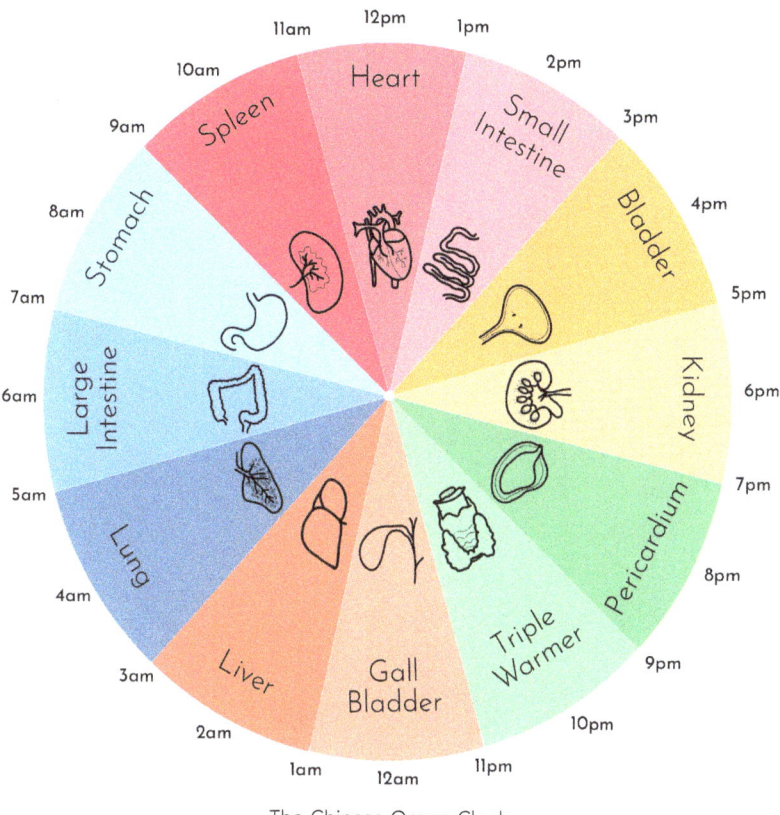

The Chinese Organ Clock

(Triple warmer, although not an actual organ,
is related to transportation of energy in the meridian system.)

The Chinese Organ Clock is an interesting part of Traditional Chinese Medicine and I find this fascinating. It is a system that describes the times of day when certain organs are at their highest and lowest levels of activity in the day and night. This may seem alien to western medicine, but it is fundamental to the concept of health and well-being in TCM. In each season, I have added the relevant times when our organs are affected for you to mull over for a bit of fun.

Emotional Freedom Technique (EFT)

EFT is one of the most advanced forms of energy psychology available to bring rapid relief to people around the world. Let me introduce you to this evidence-based and incredibly easy method of alleviating and collapsing your charged emotions and feelings.

Scientific research and evidence shows us this technique is able to reduce physical and emotional pain levels and help lessen limiting beliefs. You will feel equipped to support clients, friends and family throughout seasonal shifts.

What is it? EFT is a method of tapping with our fingers on our vital acupuncture or meridian energy points. This tapping on the meridians sends signals to the part of the brain called the hypothalamus that connects to the nervous system and in turn controls our feelings.

Our emotions can have powerful effects on our thoughts, behaviours and physical health. Whether we are feeling stressed, anxious, sad or fearful – or all these at the same time – it can lead to physical symptoms that commonly present themselves as pain or illness. EFT tapping helps clear any physical and mental symptoms by dispersing the trapped negative feeling and guiding it through the vital energy pathways for processing. It is said that our negative emotions and pain get stuck in our meridians. By gently tapping the points on the meridians these feelings reduce and disappear.

It is important to remember that emotions are like visitors: they are temporary. We can acknowledge them, and, of course, politely host them, but then say 'Bye-bye' with love and a little tapping! Guide your visitor or emotion out of the door, observe as it changes to a positive outcome after a few rounds of tapping.

EFT tapping is a brilliant tool to become healthier, happier and more balanced in the seasons. I have placed an example script at the end of each season to give you an idea of how to use it successfully yourself.

IMPORTANT FOUNDATIONS BEFORE WE BEGIN

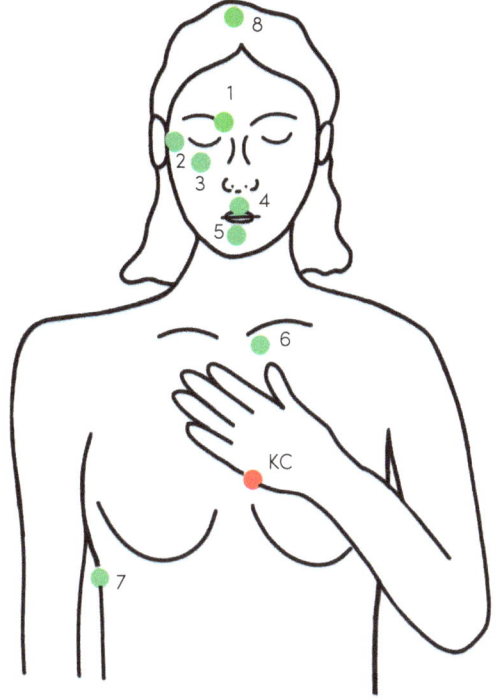

EFT focuses on nine points that are connected to a specific meridian:

1. Eyebrow (EB): bladder meridian
2. Side of the eye (SE): gall bladder meridian
3. Under the eye (UE): stomach meridian
4. Under the nose (UN): governing vessel
5. Chin (CH): central vessel
6. Beginning of the collarbone (CB): kidney meridian
7. Under the arm (UA): spleen meridian
8. Top of head (TH): governing vessel

Tapping sequence

Let's try tapping together now.

Identify the feeling or problem you would like to clear.

Rate your intensity level of the feeling or problem on a scale from zero to ten where ten is the maximum level and zero is nothing.

Using two or three fingertips on one hand, begin by tapping the side of the other hand (the karate-chop point) and repeat your set-up phrase three times. The set-up phrase acknowledges the thought or feeling you are focusing on. This could be: 'Even though I am nervous about reading this book at this time ... I deeply and completely accept myself anyway.' This phrase reminds us that we can accept ourselves even with this troubling thought or feeling.

Then, tap each point shown on the diagram above a few times, moving through the points in sequence, repeating a reminder phrase to maintain focus on your problem area, such as 'I feel sad.'

Eyebrow – I feel ...
Side of the eye – I feel ...
Under the eye – I feel ...
Under the nose – I feel ...
Chin – I feel ...
Beginning of the collarbone – I feel ...
Under the arm – I feel ...
Top of head – I feel ...

Rate the intensity of the feeling now and tap the points again until the intensity subsides.

At the end of the sequence, compare your results with your initial intensity level. If you haven't reached zero, repeat this process until you do.

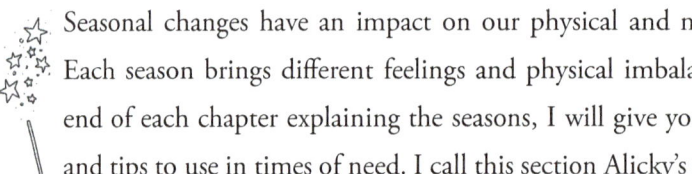 Seasonal changes have an impact on our physical and mental states. Each season brings different feelings and physical imbalances. At the end of each chapter explaining the seasons, I will give you some tools and tips to use in times of need. I call this section Alicky's magic wand.

Moments to Note in the Year

In China, the start of the seasons depends on the movements of the Moon and can fluctuate by a few weeks each year. Following the Moon means the Chinese are guided by natural forces and enjoy a fluid approach to the changes in the year. Many countries in the East celebrate the Moon cycle. Ceremonies at the time of the Full Moon are common. At this time in Sri Lanka, the temples offer a ritual of sound usings gongs and bells to clear the energy system of the body, mind and soul.

In the West, we are guided by the movement of the Earth around the Sun, which creates two solstices in the year. The word solstice means standing still.

The summer solstice is the 21st June in the northern hemisphere, and in the southern hemisphere it is the 21st December. On this day, the Sun appears to stand still as it reaches its highest point in the sky. This illusion occurs because the Earth is tilted as far as possible *towards* the Sun.

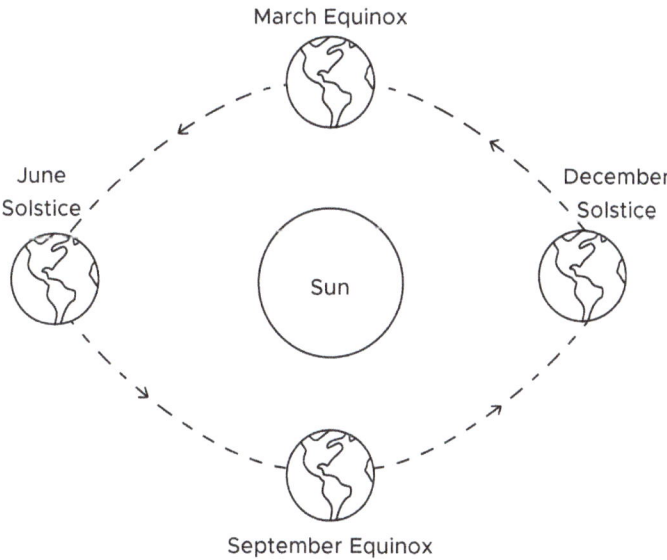

The four significant seasonal markers during the year.

The winter solstice is the 21st December in the northern hemisphere, and in the southern hemisphere it is the 21st June. The longest night of the year in the northern hemisphere is due to the Earth's axial tilt reaching its maximum distance *away* from the Sun.

The equinoxes are the only time when both the northern and southern hemisphere experience roughly equal amounts of daytime and night-time. The autumn equinox is 21st September in the north and 21st March in the south. The spring equinox is 21st March in the north and 21st September in the south.

Food

Food is our medicine. In the East, people use food and its healing properties to build up the body when deficient, cleanse it when toxic, and release the toxins when they are in excess. They sure have a lot of natural wisdom! We are now much more aware of this practice in the West, and it's become more popular to use nutrition to heal ourselves. With these simple principles of eating in harmony with the seasons, plus the awareness of the organs associated with each season and the time of day, and our changing emotions, we can all stay healthy and strong in our body, mind and spirit, with the added advantage of living long, happy and healthy lives. What's not to like about that?!

We experience food cravings when imbalanced

It seems completely normal now to eat pineapple and mangetout in winter months, but it's really not! From an energetic and environmental point of view, eating season-appropriate food is vital for our health and the health of the planet.

When we do not eat what is in season, I believe from my own learnings and wisdom that we will suffer more cravings for sweeter foods and perhaps ultra-processed foods for instant gratification. But these foods leave you feeling hungrier. It is simple to correct this, but you may need some help with tapping support because the snack cravings can also become emotional and habitual. If we are not nourished emotionally, particularly when young, we can crave foods to soothe unwanted feelings, which, of course, doesn't work in the long run. We feel more lethargic and eat more! EFT is a brilliant help for this.

Give it a go. Get in control and feel energised and empowered.

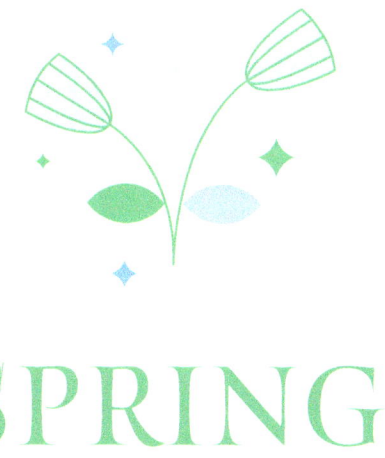

SPRING

*'No matter how long the winter is
the spring is sure to follow.'*

ANNE BRADSTREET

The Season of Spring

Months: February, March, April
Spring element: Wood
Organs: Liver and Gall Bladder
Liver and Gall Bladder active time of day: 11 p.m. to 3 a.m.

Wherever you are, the spring season is a time of new beginnings heralded by the beautiful and mood-lifting dawn chorus that strikes up at this time of year. There is a 'jump-lead effect' when you feel spring has sprung! Don't you love the carnival of scents drifting in the air and a high note of excitement as the natural world around us starts to awaken again? In spring, animals awaken from hibernation and breeding starts. Heavenly new life arrives in springtime.

Spring brings an increase in daylight, having a positive effect on our circadian rhythms, which are vital for supporting our sleep cycle. The morning light is most beneficial; morning is absolutely the best time to look up into the sky to ensure a good day ahead, so try to do this each day, whether on the way to work or just hanging out of your window for a moment or two.

Spring energy moves upwards in Chinese wisdom and can be very energising. The yang energy of the body is more masculine, strong and rising up through the body. This causes an increase in vitality and strength, which is exactly what we need after some long, dark days during the winter months.

This time is also associated with the wood element, particularly the liver aspect. This strong rising liver energy within us can also be destructive, making us feel anger and frustration, especially if we are not aligned with the energy of nature.

This is a great time for cleaning out the old to make space for the new after a long winter. So get tidying your cupboards plus your body and mind too – this will help a smooth transition through the season!

The Boons and Banes of Spring

This chart gives a brief outline of the ups and downs you may feel in springtime.

BOONS	BANES
Communication	Chaotic reactions
Positive planning	Inability to think clearly
Organised	Muddled and disorganised
Clear thought processing	Slow thought processing
New beginnings	Feeling stagnated
Emotionally balanced	Moody and frustrated

During spring, try detoxing your body and lifestyle habits, decluttering your home, and taking note of the emotions that get stirred up. Our habits are often difficult to deal with as it takes time to rewire the brain to healthier and better habits. Dealing with an addiction, such as letting go of alcohol or processed food can be difficult. Adapt the EFT tapping routine at the end of the chapter to reduce the craving for whatever you may be struggling with.

During this time, you will feel stronger, more energised, and perhaps be excited to start new projects and take action with plans that have been in the making, ready for the summer.

The Physical During Spring
Organs involved in spring: liver and gall bladder

Active times of the organ
Gall Bladder: 11 p.m. to 1 a.m.
Liver: 1 a.m. to 3 a.m.

The liver is the organ that comes into action in springtime. Energetically, the liver is the organiser within us, the planner and the master organ of detox. This amazing organ works hard to keep us clean and healthy. It filters all our unwanted toxins and any excess elements from food. Therefore, a strong, healthy and functioning liver is vital for optimal health and harmony. Western lifestyles, in particular, may cause the liver to tire and become congested with toxic overload and emotional stagnation. Keep this energy circuit of the liver open and flowing with movement, detoxification and mental cleansing.

Using the Chinese Organ Clock as our circadian rhythm guide can be extremely useful. For example, if you wake in the night between 1 a.m. and 3 a.m. your liver energy is unbalanced, perhaps in need of a detox. Waking between 11 p.m. and 1 a.m. may indicate the gall bladder energy is challenged. You also have peak times of energy in the day, this will indicate where your strengths and weaknesses are in the various organs connected to that time. As a practitioner, this knowledge vital; just for you it's a bit of informational fun. So, observe your sleep-wake patterns! Look at the foods and drink (especially alcohol) you consume, as well as the emotional aspects of the day. This will guide you to where you may be imbalanced at this time of the year.

Function of the liver

The liver is the largest solid organ in the human body and is a natural multitasker. It has a huge role to play in keeping us in tip-top shape. By following several simple steps in this chapter, we can keep our liver in good health.

The liver's key roles include:

- metabolising nutrients and removing toxins from the blood
- regulating blood sugar; converting glucose into glycogen, and storing it for future energy needs
- aiding a good immune function and fighting infection
- storing vital vitamins and minerals
- producing bile which breaks down the fats we ingest (stored in its friend the gall bladder)

From the Chinese viewpoint, the liver is associated with the element of wood. Think of trees and their strength. Rooted, strong, and always growing, maturing and flourishing. Think of the wind again. How does it affect the trees? The wind will either knock the tree over or encourage it to become stronger by developing its root structure for the next onslaught.

Imbalances of liver may lead to these physical symptoms:

- Migraines – which are due to stagnation, especially pains in the side of the head
- Vertigo and dizziness
- Stiff and painful joints
- Irritable eyes
- Heartburn and palpitations
- Hay fever

A balanced liver leads to these physical benefits:

- Clear eyes
- Good digestion
- Clear and glowing skin
- Muscular strength

Function of the gall bladder

The gall bladder stores the bile that is made by the liver. Bile is vital for breaking down fatty foods and absorbing fat-soluble vitamins.

From a Traditional Chinese Medicine point of view, the gall bladder is responsible for organisation and decision-making; also, the smooth flow of energy through the body. So, think of all those indecisive friends you have. You will now know what's going on!

Imbalances of the gall bladder may lead to these physical symptoms:

- Trouble in making decisions
- A feeling of 'stuckness'
- Struggling digestion, especially of fatty food
- Abdominal pain
- Bloating

A balanced gall bladder leads to these physical benefits:

- Strong leadership
- Effective planning
- Good digestion
- Optimal energy due to efficient nutrient absorption

The Emotional During Spring

Spring is a time for new beginnings. Both in nature and within ourselves. The energy of nature in this season is fresh and rising, so this is a great time for setting positive intentions for the year ahead. The sluggish mood we may feel from the long winter months may need to be shifted. Healing emotions for the spring are compassion, empathy and kindness, so be aware of practising these daily towards yourself and others.

The imbalance of the liver and gall bladder can bring feelings of anger, hate and jealousy adding to irritable feelings and, most annoyingly, inner conflict. Power and control are aspects of the liver energy. Too much or too little of this energy will create issues like behaving in an overbearing way, being over controlling, or even the opposite such as experiencing lack of coordination, feelings of panic or desperation. Do you recognise this?

The liver chi is very strong and can be destructive like an angry teenager! The wind can be your enemy in springtime. The Chinese masters believe the wind charges through the liver meridian, disrupting us. The toxic waste, that may be dormant from the winter months just passed, gets stirred up and rises fast, leaving us feeling unsettled, irritable and cross. We can also get itchy, weepy, yellowing eyes and hay-fever-type symptoms.

Wind helps to clear out the mental and physical heaviness left over from winter. Imagine the effect of the wind is like a large wooden spoon that comes and stirs up a murky pond that's been stagnating in the winter: all the unwanted waste, such as our unprocessed emotions, rise to the surface for filtering. So if we have nourished ourselves in winter, we shouldn't have the liver rising up to irritate us during spring!

If your liver chi is weak, the smooth flow of blood around the body may be disrupted and cause stagnation. The culprits causing these sensations are the overload of toxins that have built up through stress or poor nutrition. If we're not careful, the energy of the liver will disrupt the other carefully orchestrated energy systems too.

FEAR NOT! There is help to follow – EFT is a wonderful tool to shift and detox the mind and body.

SPRING

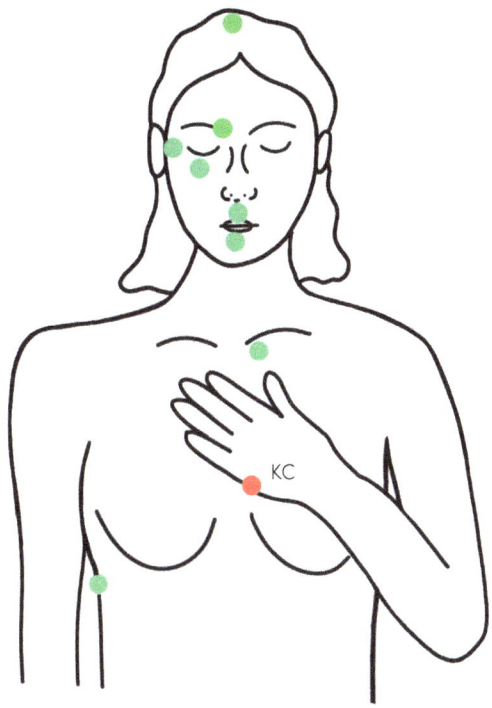

The nine points to tap when practising EFT.

EFT to Reduce Feelings of Anger, Irritability and Frustration

This is a quick script to release anger and should take roughly three minutes, depending on the level of feeling! Observe the feeling or mood that is present and taking up your headspace. Notice where you feel it most in your body. How intense is it?

1. Give the level of anger and intensity a mark first: zero (nothing at all) to ten (extreme intensity) of your feeling.

2. Take three slow, deep breaths in and out before you begin.

3. Tapping on the side of the hand (on the karate-chop point) say your set-up phrase three times as below. (We only use the karate-chop point on the side

of the hand to say the set-up statement. You can miss the karate chop point out on the subsequent rounds.)

'Even though I am angry right now, I deeply and completely accept myself anyway.'
'Even though I am angry right now, I deeply and completely accept and honour myself anyway.'
'Even though I am angry at the moment, I deeply and completely accept myself anyway, and acknowledge I feel this anger.'

4. Now, start tapping through the remaining eight points shown on the diagram above, you can start on the eyebrow, then move to the outer eye and keep going around the face and body, move from one point to the next after each line and say:

Inner eye: 'All of my anger.'
Side of eye: 'All of my anger.'
Under eye: 'I feel so angry.'
Under nose: 'I am seething.'
Chin: 'I am angry about ...'
Collar bone: 'I feel so angry.'
Under arm: 'My anger feeling.'
Top of head: 'My anger feeling.'

5. Now change the wording to start letting go in the next round following the same points as above:

'I choose to calm this anger down.'
'I choose to release this anger from every part of me.'
'It's OK to feel anger.'
'But now I choose to let it go.'
'It's OK to have this feeling of anger.'
'But now I choose to release it from my ...'

'My anger feeling in my… is calming now.'
'My anger is releasing.'

Where do you feel this anger now? Has it shifted somewhere else?

6. Next, start tapping again, guiding the mind to where the feeling is in your body. Keep tapping around the points, in the same pattern as above, and use relevant words for where you feel it now. Be aware it will move around the body and head and this is chasing it out of the physical! For example:

'My anger feeling in my tummy.'
'My anger feeling in my head.'
'My anger feeling in my chest.'

This tapping can release tears of anger and frustration, this is good news. Keep tapping around the points, shown in the diagram above, until the physical feeling has cleared.

7. If there is still some of the anger or a related feeling, such as irritation or frustration, tune into it. Tap on the remaining feeling, again moving around the points on your face and body, using words similar to these:

'My remaining anger.'
'My remaining irritation.'
'I now feel slightly sad.'
'My remaining anger.'
'My remaining irritation.'
'My remaining sadness feeling.'

Take three deep breaths, counting in for four and out for four.

8. Check your level of feeling again. Hopefully, the number has reduced dramatically. If there are any remaining feelings around your anger, then

do another round of tapping. It's OK to change the wording. Just check the emotional and physical feelings. Do you feel clearer now?

Healing emotions for the liver are compassion, empathy and kindness. Perhaps tap in some positives as well, such as:

'I have compassion for myself.'
'I choose to be kind to myself.'
'I send love and empathy to this thing I feel angry or frustrated about.'

Do this emotional tapping as many times as you would like around all the points on the body and head until you feel the benefit.

The magical world of energy is extraordinary in the way it travels unconsciously through to other people. Doing this exercise will benefit those around you as well as yourself. And in case you were wondering, you don't need to tell other people how kind you have been by sending this positive energy towards them!

Food to Nurture you in Spring

In spring, we can switch to lighter foods to detox from winter nourishment, adding in more leafy greens and vegetables that grow above ground. These vegetables are most nutrient packed in spring. They are lighter on the digestion than the root vegetables of winter. Reduce the amounts of fats you consume to give the liver and gall bladder a rest. You should also aim to eat more sour foods to enhance the liver's chi. If we are weak and out of balance, we can get ill at this time, which is an indicator of imbalance.

SPRING

FOOD TO INCLUDE

Dandelion – leaves and roots (in salads or tea, as a replacement for coffee)
Rocket
Radish
Rhubarb
Kale, spinach and nettles (with a little cheese for absorption!)
Chicken and turkey
Asparagus
Black pepper
Purple-sprouting broccoli
Pomegranate
Sesame seeds, almonds and walnuts
Magnesium-rich food
Milk thistle

Eating late can affect your digestion. If possible, eat two to three hours before bedtime, so your food can be digested and cleanse you overnight. If you wake up between 1 a.m. and 3 a.m., remember that your liver is struggling!

Drinking warm lemon and water helps to push the excess fat that your liver has not dealt with through the bowels. To prepare this drink, squeeze half to one lemon into a glass of water and drink it first thing in the morning.

RECIPES FOR SPRING

Veggie tapenade

Serves 4 to 6

Ingredients

2 tbsp. chives

1.5 cups parsley (alkaline and full of vitamin K and C)

1 cup pinenuts

1.5 cups pitted black olives

2 tbsp. capers

2 cloves garlic

1 – 2 tbsp. lemon juice

3 tbsp. olive oil

½ tsp. thyme

Black pepper

Method

Crush or blend the pinenuts. Mix all other ingredients in a blender or by hand. This tapenade can be eaten with crackers, toast or some crudites of your choice. It makes a wonderful canape. The tapenade can be kept for a few days but the nutritional value reduces the longer it is kept.

Spinach, nettle and eggs Florentine

Serves 1

Florentine means it's a dish made of spinach. This meal is particularly good in spring as the greens in this recipe support the liver and your gut as a superfood. Recommended for good health!

Ingredients

2 handfuls of spinach and nettle (wear rubber gloves to pick the youngest leaves)

2 eggs

Handful of grated parmesan (this helps absorption of the iron in the nettles and spinach)

1 tbsp. of sesame seeds (tonifies the blood and has a healthy oil content)

A liberal handful of parsley (alkaline and full of vitamins K and C)

Salt and pepper to taste

Optional extra: wild garlic and cleavers

Method

Wilt some spinach and nettle, mixed in equal quantities, in a frying pan. Nettle tastes bitter and unsavoury to some people, so I chop it up and mix it in with the spinach, and make sure to add plenty of seasoning.

Make a hole in the middle of the wilted spinach and nettle and add an egg or two.

Sprinkle some parmesan cheese on the top with some sesame seeds. I usually place a lid on the pan for a short time to melt the cheese and cook the egg faster.

Sprinkle parsley over the top with the optional extra of wild garlic and cleavers. In for a penny, in for a pound, as they say! Cleavers are a well-known weed in everyone's garden and sometimes its known fondly as 'sticky willy'. They help with inflammation and allergies, like hay fever, by clearing heat from the blood. They will also nourish the blood, which is great for the liver.

Detox salad

Serves 6

This salad is also excellent for liver health in spring and aids a detox if needed. The greens in this salad are super nutritious.

Ingredients

1 cup kale (remove very thick stalks)
1 cup nettle tops (the leaves from the top of nettle plants are less tough than the larger leaves found towards the bottom of the plant)
2 cups broccoli (good for heart health and supporting the immune system)
2 cups greens/Brussel sprouts (some greens and sprouts are cruciferous vegetables – truly fabulous for foods for your good gut bacteria)
2 cups red cabbage (a superfood rich in phytonutrients to support your immune system)
1 cup carrots (eliminates toxins and improves eye health)
½ cup fresh parsley chopped finely (alkalising for the blood and full of vitamins K and C)
½ cup almonds (high vitamin E content, so good for keeping cholesterol low)
1 to 2 tbsp. sunflower seeds (great for hypertension and headaches)
1 or 2 cups of either couscous, quinoa, brown rice or chickpeas
Seaweed is a wonderful addition but an acquired taste!

Dressing Ingredients

3 tbsp. extra virgin olive oil
½ cup lemon juice (alkalising)
1 tbsp. fresh ginger, peeled and grated (warming)
3 tsp. Dijon mustard (rich in selenium and vitamins C and A)
2 tsp. honey or maple syrup (antibacterial and antifungal)
¼ tsp. sea salt

Method

In a food processor, chop all the vegetables including the parsley and mix together in a large bowl. You will most likely have to do this in batches.

Process the almonds until roughly chopped and mix into the salad with the sunflower seeds.

Whisk the dressing ingredients together in a small bowl and drizzle over the salad.

Add couscous, quinoa, brown rice or chickpeas, which are easily digested by the liver and gall bladder and so do not put these vital organs under pressure.

Zesty rhubarb

Serves 3 to 4

Rhubarb is an excellent choice for springtime as it's abundant now. Rhubarb helps with liver congestion, mouth ulcers and cold sores. Cardamon and cinnamon help to balance the blood sugar, aid digestion and ease inflammation.

Ingredients

3 to 4 cups rhubarb, sliced into 2.5 cm pieces on a slant (antibacterial, antifungal, great for intestinal dysfunction)

¼ to ½ cup sugar (heating for the body – avoid if you are experiencing hot flushes)

Cardamon seeds crushed up (promotes circulation)

Cinnamon powder (balances blood sugar)

Zest of 1 orange

Method

Preheat oven to 175 degrees celsius.

Place sugar and orange zest in a 20 x 20 cm baking dish. Massage the sugar into the citrus zest to bring out the natural oils of the orange.

Add in rhubarb, cardamom and cinnamon and toss together.

Bake until the rhubarb is tender but not falling apart, about 25 minutes. Check halfway through and toss the contents. If the sugar is sticking to bottom of the pan, add just a teaspoon of water.

Serve with full-fat, high-protein Greek yoghurt, good-quality ice cream, or anything creamy.

Use honey or sugar to add sweetness if necessary.

Ginger, lemon and cinnamon tea

These ingredients are detoxing and anti-inflammatory, thereby aiding chronic pain which tends to be a result of inflammation – headaches are a classic example.

Slice or grate some ginger and squeeze a whole lemon into a cafetiere or teapot. If you have a cinnamon stick, add this now. If you are using cinnamon powder wait till the end to add. Steep in hot water for 5 minutes and then add a sprinkle of a little more cinnamon. If you can't bear the taste, drizzle a little honey into it to sweeten. You can also add mint to flavour the tea.

Sip throughout the day – I cover my teapot or a cafetiere with a tea cosy to keep the drink warm!

Nettle-leaf tea

Wear a pair of gloves to collect the leaves from the young nettle plant, in a clean place away from areas where dogs are walked. In Chinese medicine, nettle leaves nourish the blood and are great if you need a tonic. Nettle-leaf tea is also good for people with dry eyes, dry skin and headaches. Please remember to rinse the leaves before use.

Put a handful of roughly chopped young nettle leaves into a cafetiere or teapot of hot water.

Add few goji berries for sweetness.

Optional extra ingredients:

Dandelion and cleavers to nourish the blood and clear heat, which is great for the liver. I sometimes add mint leaves to change the flavour.

Barley water is also excellent as a detox aid (see summer recipes, p. 57).

Herbs

Herbs are an easy and effective way to add to your nutrition and support your body. Milk thistle, nettle tops (use gloves to collect), cleavers and dandelion are easily available in the West during spring and are said to help detoxify the liver in this fantastic detox season. They improve blood circulation, gastrointestinal health, reduce inflammation and boost the immune system with antiviral properties. Here are some herbal tea remedies for spring.

Alicky's Magic Wand
Exercise
Have a go at adding in jogging or some cardiovascular exercise to your routine this season. Try chi gung exercises, such as the one overleaf where swinging the body helps to detox the organs especially the liver.

Abdominal Massage Technique
This technique is wonderful to use in spring alongside a detox. This will aid any detox and help the gut to release anything you may have been holding onto, such as unwanted emotions and it helps physical digestion.

Lightly massage your abdomen clockwise, starting around the outside of your belly button, until it softens, then work outwards to the lower ribs, hip bones and pubic bone. Often you will find a stuck and solid area on your right side, just under the ribs. This indicates a congested liver. Give a little massage around the area and wait for the gurgling sound to come. That's the release of the congestion!

Fast and Detox
It's a good idea to find a detox routine that helps you, but also one that is not too harsh – there are a lot to choose from. Adding in more plant-based foods every day could help as they are packed with good nutrients. Perhaps you also need to look at adding more protein with good-quality meat (organic where possible), or pulses. I often observe that clients are not eating enough protein. Ensuring optimal protein intake helps to reduce cravings for the useless and empty calories (found in pastries, ultra-processed foods and sugar), this is because you will be getting more of the good, nutritional calories.

Intermittent fasting is a detoxing technique and lifestyle choice that works very well for some people, but remember to always get advice from an expert to guide you.

SPRING

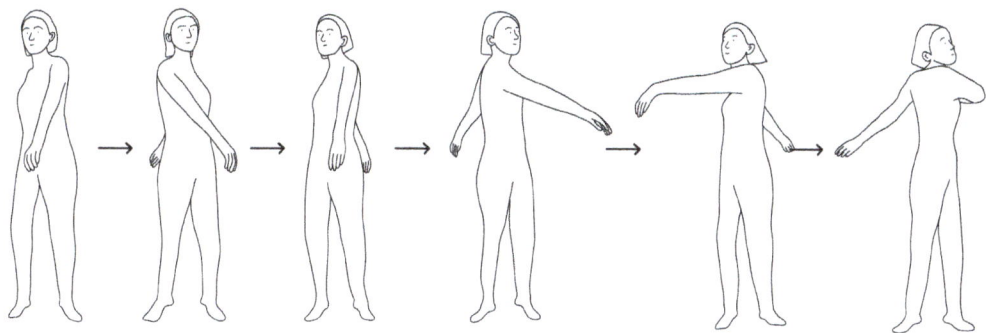

This image shows a swinging technique used in chi gung. Keeping your feet grounded, loosely swing your arms around your body starting at hip height and gradually working up to shoulder height. Move your head as your swing around.

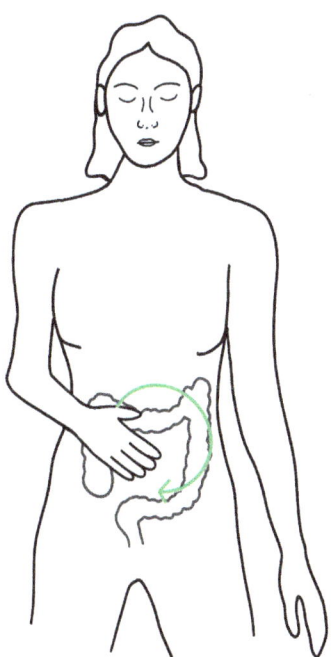

This image shows how to give yourself an abdominal massage.

Daily skin brushing

Dry brushing using a body brush is a method of detoxing that has been around for centuries. In fact, people used leaves and twigs to brush the skin in ancient times. It's believed to have many health benefits by exfoliating the skin (we detox through our skin) and it helps promote lymphatic circulation, which supports the function of detox when done regularly.

How to practise dry brushing

Start brushing at your feet and move up your body. Use light pressure in areas where your skin is thin and harder pressure on thicker skin, like the soles of your feet.

Brush your skin using a sweeping upwards motion, and don't forget your ankles. Moving up the body, brush your legs behind the knees where you have lymph glands, over your hips, abdomen and chest, sweeping outwards. Then from your hands, up your arms and finally, sweep gently up the neck.

Sage smudging and decluttering

Sage smudging is a practice that has been done for centuries to make a space more energised. A sage smudge stick is made from dried sage sprigs tied together. Sometimes thyme, mugwort and rosemary are added. The smudging ritual is a beautiful and effective technique to clear the energy and feeling in a space. You will feel lighter after each time you practise this! A smudging ritual can be done annually, once a season, or whenever you feel the need. It's especially vital to perform as part of the cleaning process when you first move into a new home. Sage is very pungent but the scent only lasts a short while, and it may be a good idea to open the windows afterwards.

Offer a sage smudge stick as a gift to a friend who has moved house to clear out the old owners' energy and bring in good energy. This is a unique gift, for sure!

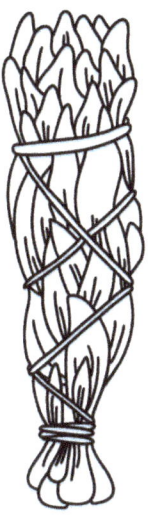

Make a smudge stick by binding together several stems of sage with string.

How to smudge the space
- Start at the front door of your home and light your smudge stick. Then, begin to move slowly around the home. Move mindfully and with care, walking clockwise around the entire interior perimeter of the building. Moving around a space like this is called circumambulation.
- Be sure to allow the smoke to drift into any hidden spaces, including inside cupboards and wardrobes, basements and dark corners. If there are stairs, just go up or down when you come across them so you can smudge the upper or lower levels in the same manner. Then keep moving clockwise around each floor until you meet the stairs again.
- When you arrive back at the front door, it's helpful to say a mantra or a prayer that is meaningful to you as a way to fill the space with more cleansing vibrations.

- Visualise the entire home filled with bright, white sunlight. Then speak your intention one last time to close the smudging ceremony. Your intention may be 'to have a happy home' or 'to have a home filled with love and abundance'.

Some example mantras to say if you so wish
- I command any negativity, any low vibrational energy that's not mine within this space, to leave. You are not welcome here. Go to the light.
- I cleanse my home of any negativity and heaviness.
- I release all attachment to the negative or unwanted energy that has invaded my space and choose freedom and light.
- I release any worry from my body and my home.
- I welcome positivity, love and joy into my home.
Have a go and enjoy!

If you can't bear the smoke, an alternative to smoky smudging is making a mist spray combining the essential oils of Palo Santo or white sage, water and a little white spirit in a clean spray bottle. Spray regularly around the space as above instructions.

Gardening

Gardening is well known to raise the emotional bar with its microbial properties released as we dig in the fresh air. You can plant vegetables and flowers outside in pots or in the ground. Think of clean home-grown veggies, no additives, no pesticides and the pleasure of creating your own nutrition – but beware of those pesky late spring frosts! Inside, you can still experience the benefit by growing green plants in your house to bring in fresh energy from nature.

Meditation

The word meditation used to send all the wrong signals for me. Sitting crossed legged on a floor (not happening!) and emptying your mind – what? No way is that going to happen!

SPRING

If someone had said: take a quiet moment, close your eyes, and observe what you feel, hear and smell – I would have got it straight away. So, therefore, I invite you to do the same.

Take a moment to think about what and how you feel as the spring season comes in and then goes out again into summer. Note this down. Take three deep breaths right down into the bottom of your lungs and slowly release each breath. I usually do some tapping at this stage if I have sensed an imbalance, tightness or worry.

MANTRA
'I choose to embrace life as it comes.'

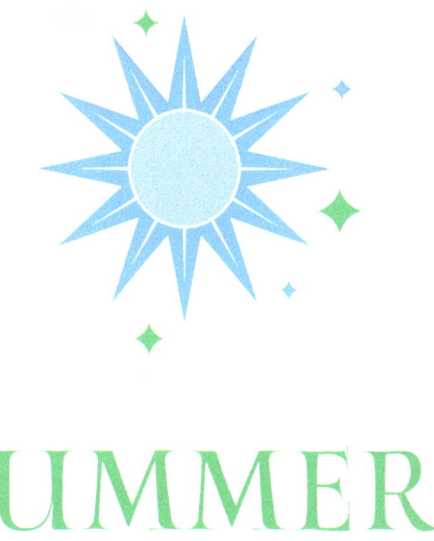

SUMMER

*'The earth does not belong to us.
We belong to the earth.'*
Chief Seattle of the Suquamish Tribe

The Season of Summer

Months: May and June (early summer), July and August (late summer)
Summer element: Fire and Earth
Organs: Heart, Small Intestine, Stomach, and Spleen
Stomach and Spleen active time of day: 7 a.m. to 11 a.m.
Heart and Small Intestine active time of day: 11 a.m. to 3 p.m.

In Chinese wisdom, and it is increasingly understood in the western cultures, the summer is split into two parts: early summer and late summer or high summer and low summer.

Summer energy expands outwards. According to Chinese wisdom, the unique energies of early summer influence the heart and small intestine. Late summer energy influences the stomach and spleen.

The summer months are a time for socialising, celebrating and connecting. The summer brings laughter, lightness, and generally, more joy than the dark winter months. We spend more time outside socialising late into the warmer evenings – forever hopeful of good weather in the northern hemisphere!

The heart is the ruler or governor of our energetic system and houses the spirit within us. Its job and function is to oversee the workings of the mind, body and spirit. Our heart is sacred, so my advice is to look after it well.

The heart also governs the arteries and is therefore in charge of circulation. We would die if the heart stops beating and circulating our blood. The small intestine oversees the absorption of nutrients coming into your sacred body, separating the important nutrition and waste from your food. Vitally, it helps keep us toxin free and keeps our energy high and positive in summertime.

As late summer approaches, the Earth energy, which influences the spleen and stomach, becomes more active to provide nourishment to the body and soul. The spleen and stomach aid in the absorption of nutrients and the smooth flow of energy and blood. If the energy of these organs is weak then we may worry excessively, brood over emotions and overthink.

The Boons and Banes of Summer

This chart gives a brief outline of the ups and downs of your feelings in summertime.

BOONS	BANES
Celebration	Worry
Joy	Confusion and brain fog
Compassion	Cravings for sweet foods
Higher energy levels	Unsettled and restless
Feeling settled	Overwhelm
Balance	Moody and frustrated

The Physical During Early Summer

Organs involved in early summer (May and June): heart and small intestine

Active times of the organs

Heart and small intestine: 11 a.m. to 3 p.m.

This period of active times for early summer organs may be your high energy time of day if you are balanced. If there are physical issues with your heart or small intestine, you might feel at your lowest energy during this time of the day.

The heart energy, with all its emotional connections, is our life force and beats in order to move blood, oxygen and nutrients to the cells around the body.

Physical imbalances in the heart may lead to:

- Heart palpitations
- Shortness of breath
- Sweating and overheating

A balanced heart leads to these physical benefits:

- Good circulation
- Increased energy levels
- Well-regulated body temperature

The small intestine starts the vital process of breaking down food, sorting out the good nutrients from the bad stuff, and removing these unwanted toxic invaders. The small intestine assists the function of the heart by purifying and transporting fluids and substances that enter the blood stream.

Physical imbalances in the small intestine may lead to:

- Digestive disturbance
- Low physical energy

A balanced small intestine leads to these physical benefits:

- Good digestion and absorption
- Higher physical energy

The Emotional During Early Summer

If we are in balance, the heart energy conveys love and kindness. A fascinating fact is that kindness hormones such as oxytocin present themselves when you show kindness. Someone who talks about this is Dr Tara Swart, I have huge admiration for this leading neuroscientist and author of one of my favourite books – *The Source*. A touch, hand hold or kiss on the cheek from a loved one or friend activates the release of oxytocin in both participants. Therefore, one surmises that being loving and kind can lower the risk of heart problems significantly. How lovely is that to hear! If we experience an emotional imbalance in early summer, it can bring up feelings where there is a lack of kindness and love, instead there is sadness and grief. People with low heart chi or energy can be unkind in nature and lack emotional regulation. With too much heart chi they can be loud and opinionated.

When balanced, the small intestine purveys clarity and feeling connected. The energy of a balanced small intestine protects the spirit of the heart by filtering out negative elements. I view the small intestine as a traffic controller, supporting the decision around what is allowed in and what is not – both physically and energetically, like the Hogwarts sorting hat! If this sorting function is not operating efficiently, there will be confusion in the body and mind, which can manifest as trouble with hearing, digestion and decision-making.

The Shen or Spirit

The heart also is the energetic home of the spirit or shen in Chinese medicine. As an organ in western wisdom, it is the supreme governor of the body. We wouldn't be alive if we lost our heart. Through the heart we are energetically closest to the deepest source of our being.

This is why trainers and gurus of healing principles will always ask you to connect into your breath and take it down to your heart. Joy, happiness and intimacy, but also sadness, is felt in our heart. In western medicine the language around the heart is interesting. The words 'faint-hearted, half-hearted, good-hearted' all give us clues. 'Heartbreak' is a phenomenon seen by cardiologists: literally, the heart cracks and this is called Broken Heart Syndrome (as explained in the book *The Five Side Effects of Kindness* by Dr David Hamilton, a leading expert in the science of kindness and its impact on human health).

The Physical During Late Summer
Organs involved in late summer (July and August): stomach and spleen

Active times of the organs
Stomach and spleen: 7 a.m. to 11 a.m.

These organs become more energetic later in summer and are crucial for the digestion and assimilation of food because they also separate what we need and don't need, physically and mentally.

The spleen is one of the most important organs in TCM as it is in charge of extracting the vital energy (chi) we need from food and transporting it in truck loads to all the vital areas. In western terms we can live without our spleen as other organs will adapt physically to its absence. But its energetic meridian stays with us even if we do not have the spleen.

The stomach receives nourishment, integrating and passing on broken down foods to the intestines for distribution. The stomach pulls the chi from foods. If it is not functioning, there will be weakness and lethargy. The sayings 'I cannot stomach this information' and 'I cannot take this in' refer to the mental inability to assimilate information.

The stomach and spleen are active in the morning; time for breakfast in any season. The assimilation process is active and at its best now. If your stomach and spleen are out of balance and struggling, you will feel sluggish emotionally and physically during this time of the day.

Physical imbalances in the stomach may lead to:

- Digestive issues
- Nausea or vomiting if the wrong foods are ingested and are unable to support the system

A balanced stomach leads to this physical benefit:

- Good digestion and absorption

Physical imbalances in the spleen may lead to:

- Fatigue and feeling cold, especially in the early afternoon
- Food cravings, especially for sweet food
- Weight gain
- Water retention

A balanced spleen leads to these physical benefits:

- Lean body
- Good easy digestion
- No cravings

The Emotional During Late Summer

The emotional imbalances in late summer can come to us through worry, overthinking, a lack of joy and neediness. We may feel unable to receive love or be nurtured, which so many of us struggle with accepting. The stomach and spleen are connected to being emotionally supported and loved, especially when we are young. Therefore, we may feel an extra need for love and nurture during this time. This is the perfect time of year to balance these emotions, clear any lack if we feel it, and prevent excessive feelings returning. Healing emotions in the summer are support and self-love.

EFT to Reduce Feelings of Lack of Joy

This is a quick script to release any lack of joy you might be feeling if your emotions are imbalanced in summer. You can adapt this script for other concerns, such as food cravings. It should take roughly three minutes, depending on the level of feeling!

Observe the feelings or thoughts that might be taking up your headspace right now. Choose the strongest thought or feeling and give it a title, in this case

SUMMER

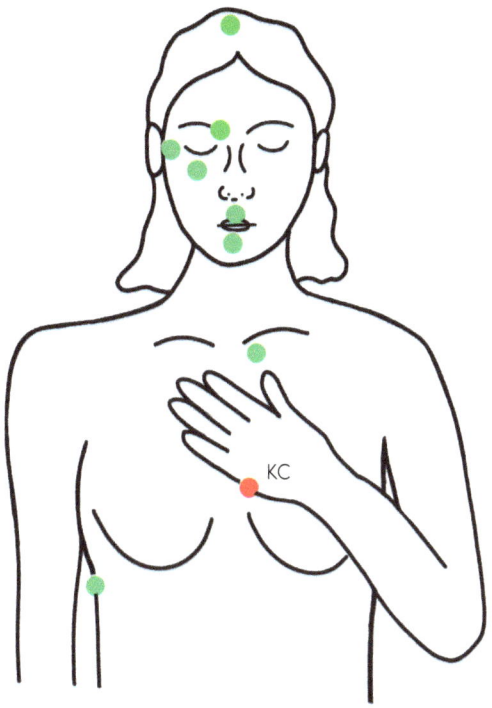

The nine points to tap when practising EFT.

'lack of joy'. Make a note of your mood or feelings around a lack of joy. Then, check the intensity of your feeling.

Take lack of joy as an example:

1. Give the level of intensity of the feeling of 'lack of joy' a mark: zero (nothing at all) to ten (extreme intensity) of your feeling.

2. Take three slow, deep breaths in and out before you begin.

3. Tapping on the side of the hand, on your karate-chop point, say your set-up phrase three times as below. (We only use the karate-chop point on the side of the hand to say the set-up statement.)

'Even though I am feeling a lack of joy right now, I deeply and completely accept myself anyway.'

'Even though I am feeling a lack of joy right now, I deeply and completely accept and honour myself anyway.'

'Even though I am feeling a lack of joy at the moment, I deeply and completely accept myself anyway, and acknowledge I feel this feeling.'

4. Then, tap through each of the points in the diagram, starting on the eyebrow point then move to the outer eye. Keep tapping around the face and body back up to the top of head point. Move from one point to the next after each script line and say:

Inner eye: 'I feel no joy.'
Side of eye: 'I feel no joy.'
Under eye: 'I feel no joy.'
Under nose: 'I feel no joy.'
Chin: 'I have no joy because ...' (e.g. I am lonely.)
Collar bone: 'I feel no joy.'
Under arm: 'My lack of joy.'
Top of head: 'My lack of joy feeling.'

5. Now change the wording in the next round, to start letting go. Tap around the points in the same order as above and choose one of the statements below. You may find a few of these resonate with you or you could use them one at a time:

'I choose to feel joyful and let go of the old feeling.'
'I choose to feel joy in every part of me.'
'I don't need this lack feeling anymore.'
'I now choose to let it go.'
'I don't need this lack of joy feeling.'
'It's OK to have this feeling sometimes.'
'But now I choose to release it from my heart.'

Where do you feel lack feeling now? Has it shifted somewhere else?

6. Next, start tapping again, guiding the mind to where the feeling is in your body. It will move around if you focus on it, so use the relevant words to direct your mind towards it and tap around the points in the same sequence. For example:

'This feeling in my tummy.'
'This feeling in my head.'
'This feeling in my chest.'
'Now I feel it in my neck.'

This tapping can release tears, connected to this feeling and this is good news. Keep tapping until the tears have cleared. You can also experience a feeling of exhaustion temporarily or yawn excessively. This is also known as clearing the emotion!

7. Now, tune into the feeling again. It may have changed to another feeling and that's also good. So use the words relevant to the feeling. Tap on this remaining feeling with words that may be similar to these:

'My remaining feeling.'
'My remaining emotion.'
'I now feel joy coming back into my whole being.'

Take three deep breaths, counting in for four and out for four.

8. Check your level of feeling again. Hopefully, the number has reduced dramatically. If there are any remaining feelings around your lack of joy and other thoughts coming up then do another round of tapping. It's OK to change the wording. Just check the emotional and physical feelings. Do you feel clearer now?

After each round, take a deep breath. Tune into how that feeling is now. Is it real? Has the feeling evaporated? If the feeling of intensity is still there, then tap again starting at the eyebrow point. Perhaps there is a reason the joy is lacking? Use the words as they come up, for example, 'My lack of joy is because I am lonely.' You are free to tap on the word 'lonely' instead.

At the end of the process, hold your hands over your heart and take three slow, deep breaths while focusing on your heart area. Know that when you're feeling clear it will help others too as the energy clearing is shared widely! It's magical stuff! So, it's interesting to observe how the people you are close to are feeling when you have finished tapping.

This completes the session.

Food to Nurture you in Summer

In summertime, we can eat more raw foods than at other times of the year because they have a cooling effect on the body rather than a warming one. If you find you cannot digest raw salads and vegetables, and you experience bloating or indigestion, then warm the food by stir frying or steaming. In summer, be careful to avoid heavy meals and excess food intake. This will exhaust your system during the season when you want to be most active and productive.

FOOD TO INCLUDE
Naturally sweet foods – honey
Berries
Pineapple (particularly good for clearing heat out of the body)
Sesame seeds
Cereals like millet and barley
Cucumber
Dark chocolate
Spices such as cardamom and cloves (lower the risk of heart disease)
Mint

RECIPES FOR SUMMER

Cold cucumber and mint soup

Serves 3 to 4

This soup is cool and refreshing on a hot day, a brilliant recipe for when the Sun decides to show its face. If you tend to become hot quickly, this soup is ideal for you. Cucumbers are surprisingly nutritious, easy to grow and have a high water content. It is said that cucumbers help reduce blood sugar and counter constipation due to their fibre content.

You can freeze the soup, but don't add the yoghurt before freezing, instead mix it in at the last minute before serving.

Ingredients

1 large cucumber, peeled and diced (vitamin K)
6 spring onions (great for any stomach upsets)
250 ml chicken stock or water (supports gut microbiome)
3 tbsp. good-quality high-protein Greek yoghurt or homemade kefir
1 lemon, squeezed (alkalising for the body)
6 sprigs of fresh mint (cooling for the eyes and head)
Salt and pepper

Method

Blend the cucumber and spring onions and water or stock together.
Add yoghurt and lemon juice and a few chopped mint leaves to garnish.
Put in fridge for one hour before serving.

Chilled summer salad

Serves 6

This salad is lovely in summer and I like to eat it with some fresh fish or chicken.

Ingredients

6 tomatoes (includes lysine)

2 small cucumbers (vitamin K)

1 courgette – grated (sweet tasting and helps clear excess heat from the body)

4 radishes (vitamin C, can help reduce phlegm, microbial boosting spicy flavour)

2 spring onions (great for any stomach upsets)

1 large gherkin (beneficial gut food)

1 large pepper (circulates blood, disperses cold from the body)

½ cup green olives (eliminates toxins)

½ cup red onion (quercetin has anti-inflammatory and antihistamine properties)

½ cup fresh parsley (cleansing)

3 tbsp. extra virgin olive oil (great superfood all year round!)

1–2 tbsp. lemon juice (alkalising)

Salt and pepper

Method

Chop and dice all ingredients to your liking. Toss into a large bowl and stir. Allow salad to marinate for one hour in the fridge. Remember, eating cooler foods during the summer is good!

Chinese sesame seed cookies

Makes approx 15

This is an excellent sweet treat and will balance the energy of the stomach and spleen. Do not eat these in a great quantity as they will promote dampness and heat in the body, which we don't want!

Ingredients

2 cups sesame (nourishes blood and chi and has healthy oil content)

2 tbsp. melted butter

¼ cup local honey or manuka

1 tbsp. sesame oil

1 tsp. vanilla (good gut soother)

½ tsp. cinnamon (balances blood sugars)

Method

Dry roast the sesame seeds until a strong aroma rises. (DO NOT BURN!) Grind them up and stir in all the other ingredients. Press the mixture together and keep cool. Shape the mixture into small marble-sized balls using wet hands. Serve on a pretty plate, to further enhance your summer joy!

Herbs

Add some herbs to your food. Rocket, parsley, mint, dill, tarragon, rosemary, lemon balm, thyme and basil all grow abundantly in summer. Try growing herbs in pots or even between flowers in a border.

Tea remedy for summer

Green tea is useful for cooling and aids digestion if you are sluggish in mind and tummy! Loose-leaf tea is probably best, but use whatever you can find. Drink a cup after a meal to help with the breakdown of food. Add a teaspoon of local or manuka honey for a slightly sweeter taste if you want.

Digestion soother

The ingredients in this tea are all wonderful for your digestion, which possibly will be sluggish at this time of year. Packed with minerals, these herbs will help with your digestion, relieve breathing ailments and improve alertness in your brain.

Ingredients

1 tsp. freshly chopped or dried basil (balances energy and disperses phlegm)
1 tsp. freshly chopped or dried mint (cooling)
1 tsp. aniseed (helps reduce flatulence)

Method

Infuse in boiled water for 5 minutes and drink up!

SUMMER

Barley water (This is helpful all year round)

Barley water is reputedly a secret weapon for good health, as it is refreshing, soothing and strengthening, especially during convalescence. It is a great aid for detoxing.

Method

Dry roast a cup of barley for 10–15 minutes in a hot oven or on the hob. Add a litre of water and bring to a slow boil on the hob for 15 minutes. Lower heat and simmer for 30–40 minutes until the barley is soft and disintegrating. Strain the barley, discard and add a little fresh lemon juice to the liquid.

The barley water can be diluted or drunk neat. Honey can be added, but I would suggest drinking without honey to reduce blood sugar spikes. Also, I recommend drinking this in the morning before breakfast.

Alicky's Magic Wand
Exercise

Dancing is a good activity for the summer months when your energy is high and you need to remain active. Zumba, salsa, or even line dancing – whatever makes you happy! Dancing around in the garden at sundown after a glass of wine (or two) makes me happy! Cycling and going on a fast walk are also effective at keeping your energy active.

Another good technique that helps to balance and open the energy up through your meridian channels is a good stretch. Sit on a blanket (preferably outside) and bring the soles of your feet together. Lie back, arms out wide. Inhale and exhale into your abdomen.

HeartMath breathing

This breathing technique regulates your heart rate variability (HRV). When we are stressed or anxious our HRV becomes disrupted, causing heart palpitations and feelings of anxiety. HeartMath breathing works by focusing your attention in the area of the heart and imagining your breath is flowing in and out of your heart or chest area, breathing a little slower and deeper than usual. Inhale for five seconds, then exhale for five seconds (or whatever rhythm is comfortable).

Rib rubbing

Consider adding some gentle massage, such as rubbing the area under your breasts to active good spleen energy. Or rub the outer corner of the knee to activate and soothe the stomach.

Feel love

Spend time with loved ones who you admire, and they will radiate positive energy towards you. You know the ones I am talking about!

Walk in nature

Walk mindfully, while the ground is warm and hopefully dry. Be aware of each of your senses – sight, hearing, smell and touch – while you walk.

Thumb holding

When anxiety strikes or you feel nervous energy inside, hold your thumb with the opposite hand. Wait till you feel a pulse in the thumb. This indicates the energy flow and switches on a calming feeling. Think of babies sucking their thumbs to soothe themselves – they have the knowledge unconsciously.

Journalling

Write down your worries anywhere – a scrap of paper or a journal will be fine. If this makes you feel emotional, don't forget you can do some EFT tapping to help! It is also important to trust that these worries will pass. Make a note about what you love about yourself and what you are offering in this world right now. Put the note somewhere you will see this daily to remind yourself.

Gratitude

Be supremely grateful for any joy in your day. Before I go to sleep, I say my thanks for the positive events in the day, such as a delicious coffee, the sunshine, or a kind gesture from someone. This concentrates the brain on these joyful moments while you are sleeping rather than the irritating stuff experienced in the day which we can ruminate over at night.

Laughter

Watch funny movies to keep the heart energy raised.

MANTRA

Summer mantra to say before sleep and on waking:
'I appreciate and love who I am.'

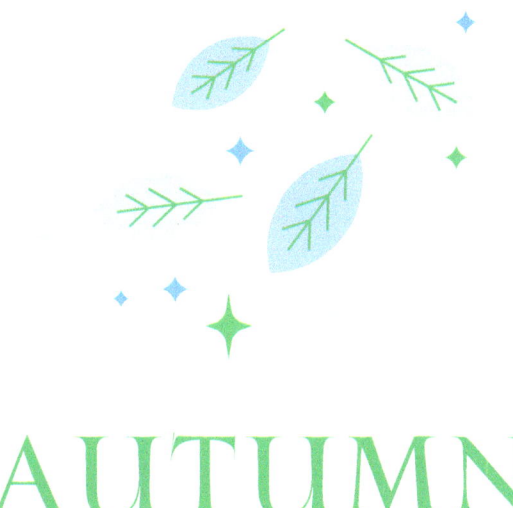

AUTUMN

*'Autumn teaches us the beauty of letting go.
Growth requires release. It is what the trees do.'*
Ka'ala

The Season of Autumn

Months: September, October, November
Autumn element: Metal
Organs: Lungs and Large Intestine
Lungs and Large Intestine active time of day: 3 a.m. to 7 a.m.

When the long days of summer take their final bow, autumn often appears quite suddenly. These three months of the year are a great time for self-development and consolidating the year's learnings. It is a time to retreat, to create some inner peace and harmony. Autumn energy moves downwards in the body and in nature as plants fade into the earth to regenerate for spring. Trees lose their leaves to restore the vitality of the tree within. Bountiful crops are harvested during autumn.

Autumn is a time for storing the vital chi in our bodies for the winter months ahead. It is known as a time for contraction and moving inward. Therefore, the energy focus of this season shifts to our inner relationship with ourselves after our expansive energy in the summer months. If we don't follow this wisdom, we can become weak during the autumn, carry this through to winter and struggle in the following year.

This season is connected to the lungs and large intestine. Possible bowel or lung problems will show up now – we all experience that autumn cold, cough and virus each year.

I always feel that autumn is a better time for starting to reset your path rather than the new year in January. It is a key time for creating routine and stability to build on later.

I feel autumn is a time to release our unwanted guests – thoughts, draining relationships and unhealthy habits – and taking the time to look at any workload you may have. Breath exercises are key during this time, as keeping our lungs energised prepares us for the long, harsh winter ahead.

The Boons and Banes of Autumn

This chart gives a brief outline of the ups and downs of your feelings in autumn time.

BOONS	BANES
Time for regrouping, consolidating	Less daylight
Slowing down in line with nature	Withdrawing and loneliness
Showing vitality in body and mind	Constipation or diarrhoea
Consolidating and reflecting on the year's learnings	Sadness and Seasonal Affective Disorder (SAD)
Inspirational time for new ideas	Lack of creativity

The Physical During Autumn

This section provides an overview of how the body responds in autumn.

Organs involved in autumn: lungs and large intestines

Active times of the organs

Lungs: 3 a.m. to 5 a.m.

Large intestine: 5 a.m. to 7 a.m.

Functions of the lungs and large intestine

We take around 25,000 breaths a day! The lungs take in oxygen and transfer it to your bloodstream to be transported around the body. On the out breath, the lungs expel carbon dioxide and any unwanted toxic waste from the air to stop them entering our bloodstream.

The large intestine is the last organ of the digestion process. The last ten per cent of the process to absorb our vitamins and water happens here. The function of this organ is vital for the final formation of unwanted toxic material to be evacuated.

The intestine is made of neural tissue, which is the same as brain tissue. Therefore, due to this connection to the brain, it is important to keep this miraculous organ working well and healthy for optimal mental health too. The brain and intestine are connected by the vagus nerve, see the section below.

In eastern understanding, the lungs energetically rule the exterior of the body – the skin – through which air, water vapour and chi are exchanged. This process links lung health to skin health.

The large intestine is all about 'letting go' of emotions and old painful experiences. Think of the evacuation of waste through your bowel movements: the emotions are the same, and they need to be released.

Physical imbalances of the lungs and large intestine may lead to:

- bad, rancid breath
- intestinal cramping, rumblings and blockages
- shortness of breath, tightness in the chest
- asthma
- eczema and skin rashes
- dry lips

Getting exercise in the morning is particularly important in autumn, although beneficial in all seasons, as daylight hours decrease. Morning light creates lightness in your day and helps to reset your circadian rhythm, your wake/sleep cycle. Morning light also helps push aside the heaviness of seasonal affective disorder (SAD syndrome), which can creep in as the autumn darkness starts to take hold. Regular bowel movements are important to avoid wind or bloating. Strive for lightness and determination in your mood.

In western culture, the connection between the large intestine and the brain is thought to be via the vagus nerve. Keeping our large intestine in good health through everything we ingest and making sure the gut microbiome is supported and well-nourished will have an extremely positive impact on our mental health.

Balanced lungs and large intestine lead to these physical benefits:

- Good wake/sleep cycle
- Regular bowel movements
- Efficient digestion
- Great vitality

Vagus nerve

Although it has been known for decades, only recently has the mind–body and gut–brain connection become more well researched, widely believed and now even fashionable.

The brain, heart and gut are connected by something we call the vagus nerve. The discovery of this vagus nerve has proved that the mind-body connection, which has long been discussed in traditional Chinese wisdom, is true. What the mind presents is often what is going on in the body, especially the gut. The happy hormone, serotonin, is produced in the gut, which not only makes us happy, but also lowers stress by regulating the central nervous system and calming the heart.

The Emotional During Autumn

Emotional imbalance, which sometimes comes out as SAD in autumn, is a common issue for lots of people as the light fades and the days shorten. A feeling of detachment holding you back from life may appear as sadness, grief, low mood and depression, leaving you with a lack of self-esteem and enthusiasm, along with an inability to set proper boundaries.

When you are in emotional balance, you wake up feeling bright and energised for the day ahead. You feel emotionally well and strong and are rested and nourished. There will be an admiration and respect for others. It is vital to find something that gives you purpose every day.

As mentioned, in eastern thinking the autumn is key to creating routine and stability for the following year. Have a think about what routines you need to create for yourself to find some purpose.

Qualities of people with strong lungs and a healthy large intestine include being hard workers, trustworthy, and dependable. They will always be able to finish a project; they may even be the strong silent type.

Some downfalls of weak lungs and large intestine can result in difficulties in close relationships, not allowing shared thoughts or feelings, feeling lonely and misunderstood, and a tendency to feeling blue and sad.

Autumn is a time of contraction and cooling: moving inward. It is a time to let go of old grief and unwanted patterns. This time is certainly not to be ignored and skipped over. Honour yourself by allowing a few minutes a day to tap or breathe deeply, especially while out in the autumnal morning light.

EFT to Reduce Feelings of Sadness or Low Energy

This is a quick script to release sadness and should take roughly three minutes, depending on the level of feeling! Sadness can also turn to feelings of guilt when we start tapping so keep an open mind.

Make a note of any low energy or feelings of sadness and choose the feeling that resonates with you now. Observe the feeling or mood that is present and taking up your headspace. Give the feeling a title e.g. 'sadness', and check the intensity of your feeling. Notice where you feel it most in your body.

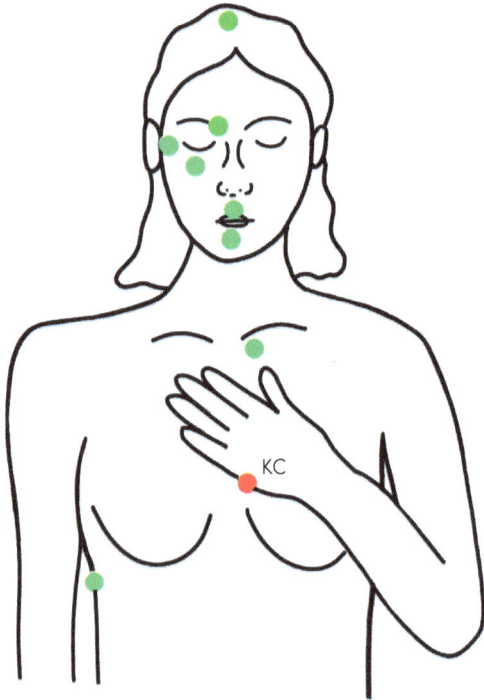

The nine points to tap when practising EFT.

1. Give the level of sadness and intensity a mark first: zero (nothing at all) to ten (extreme intensity) of your feeling.

2. Take three slow, deep breaths in and out before you begin.

3. Tapping on the side of the hand, on the karate-chop point, say your set-up phrase three times as below. (We only use the karate-chop point on the side of the hand to say the set-up statement. You can miss the kareate chop point out on subsequent rounds.)

'Even though I am feeling sad right now, I deeply and completely accept myself anyway.'

'Even though I am feeling sad right now, I deeply and completely accept and honour myself anyway.'

'Even though I am feeling sad at the moment, I deeply and completely accept myself anyway, and acknowledge I feel this sadness.'

4. Then start tapping through the points on the face and body shown in the diagram, starting on the eyebrow point, move from one point to the next after each script line and say:

Inner eye: 'All of my sadness.'
Side of eye: 'All of my sadness.'
Under eye: 'I feel so sad.'
Under nose: 'I am sad.'
Chin: 'I am sad about ... (e.g. losing someone, or just sad because ...)'
Collar bone: 'I feel so sad.'
Under arm: 'My sadness I feel.'
Top of head: 'My sadness.'

5. Now change the wording to start letting go of this feeling in the next round. You may have one feeling remaining so tap on that with a full round of points. Or if you have a few feelings coming up then you may want to stay here and tap them out too. There is no hurry. Tap around the points in the same sequence as above starting with the inner eyebrow:

'I choose to let this sadness go.'
'I choose to release this sadness from every part of me.'
'It's OK to feel sad.'
'But now I choose to let it go.'
'It's OK to have this feeling of sadness.'
'But now I choose to release it from my ...' (wherever it may be in the body.)

Where do you feel this sadness now? Has it shifted somewhere else?

6. Next, start tapping again, guiding the mind to where the feeling is in your body. Keep tapping around the points in the same pattern as above using relevant words. Where do you feel it now? It can move around the body and head so be aware! This is chasing the feeling out of the physical body. For example:

'This sadness in my tummy.'
'This sadness in my head.'
'This sadness all around me.'
'In my chest.'

This tapping can release tears of sadness too and this is good news. Keep tapping until the physical and emotional feeling has cleared.

7. Now, tune into the feeling again. It may have changed to another feeling and that's also good. So use the words relevant to the feeling. Tap on this remaining feeling with words that may be similar to these:

'My remaining sadness.'
'My remaining sadness.'
'My remaining sadness all around me.'
'I now feel better, lighter and clearer.'

Take three deep breaths, counting in for four and out for four.

8. Check your level of feeling again. Hopefully, the number has reduced dramatically. If there are any remaining feelings around your sad feeling, then do another round of tapping. It's OK to change the wording. As I have said before, just check the emotional and physical feelings. Do you feel clearer now? Perhaps tap in some positives for the healing to increase. Move around the points again, starting at the inner eyebrow.

AUTUMN

'I have compassion for myself.'
'I choose to let go of this stuck feeling with love and the wisdom I have gained.'
'I choose to nourish my mind, body and soul at this time.'

Observe the changes you notice in yourself, particularly the following day. Is your sleep better? Maybe you have more energy, or feel more grounded as a result of your EFT tapping. It is powerful and magical, so don't underestimate the changes you can make in a short time. This completes the session.

Food to Nurture you in Autumn

Our dopamine levels need boosting at this time of year as the light fades. Choose wisely and think about how you feel when you ingest certain foods. Do they make you feel energised, bloated, blocked or fulfilled? Taking time to do this in this closing season will bring you in tune with which foods may suit you. Think about what is growing in the garden and the fields. Focus meals around the foods that are in season locally and others in the table below.

FOOD TO INCLUDE
Warm stews, especially with beef
Salty and moisturising food
Rice
Pumpkins
Beef or vegetable broth
Cinnamon and cloves
Chillies and peppers
Avocados
Apples and pears, especially poached
Garlic

RECIPES FOR AUTUMN

Honey garlic

This recipe has antiviral and antibacterial properties to support our immune system as we move into autumn

Ingredients

One pot of local honey (this is important as local honey is unlikely to have been heat-treated and is full of local-flora goodness), or use manuka honey from New Zealand that is graded in strength and known for its high levels of antiviral and antibiotic properties.

Many garlic cloves – aim to fill half a jar with crushed garlic.

Method

Squish the garlic gloves slightly and half fill an empty jar.

Pour in the honey. The honey should fill the jar to the top. Seal the jar with no air gap if possible. Turn daily for six weeks.

This garlic honey is super potent and a wonderful addition to meals and marinades. Use it in dressings for salads or vegetables, or just take a tablespoon daily when feeling under the weather.

Egg nori soup

Serves 2 to 4

Seaweed and shitake mushrooms are revered in the eastern world for their famous medicinal qualities. This nurturing soup creates a deep and earthy flavour containing lots of iodine and calcium contributing to your good health. It is said this soup will help purify the blood and relieve congestion in the airways.

Ingredients

6 shitake mushrooms (if dried then soak for 10 minutes before using)

1 small leek (good for the heart)

1 cup fresh chopped-up nettles and/or seaweed/nori (great detoxifying weeds)

1 small carrot (for good eye health)

2 tsp. fresh ginger (for warming the body)

2 tbsp. soy sauce

4 cups water

2 eggs (good source of protein and they nourish the blood)

Toasted sesame oil

Method

Chop the mushrooms into thin slices.

Finely chop the leek, nettles/seaweed, carrot and ginger. Add to a pan with the water and bring to the boil.

Add soy sauce and continue boiling until the liquid has reduced by a third.

Beat the eggs in a small bowl.

Stir the soup until you create a whirlpool. Pour the eggs in so that they form long strands.

Add a drizzle of sesame oil and soy sauce and serve immediately.

Baked pears with juniper

Serves 4

Pears are abundant at this time and are a powerhouse of vitamins and antioxidants helping blood pressure and cholesterol. Combined with honey this recipe is great for cleansing any toxicity out of the body and has a mild laxative effect.

Ingredients

8 ripe pears (can clear phlegm)
6 tbsp. apple juice, made fresh in a juicer if possible (packed with polyphenols for your gut health)
1 tbsp. lemon juice (alkalising)
½ tsp. crushed coriander seeds (strengthens digestion)
8 juniper berries (diuretic effect on the body)
Honey to taste (antibacterial and antifungal))
Optional: Yoghurt to serve (good gut food)
A sprinkle of flaked almonds (high nutrient content)

Method

Halve the pears and put in a baking dish with a lid.

Cover with apple and lemon juice, sprinkle the coriander and juniper seeds over the pears.

Bake at 200 degrees celsius for about 30 minutes.

Serve with honey, yoghurt and toasted almonds. A few leaves of mint crushed up and pinch of cinnamon can be a nice addition.

Herbs

Herbs can be used to help our circulation and prepare for the colder weather. Autumn is a time when we tend to become sick with lung issues, but herbs can be a great support to our immune function.

Try adding the following herbs and spices to meals or in hot drinks:

- Hawthorn – a valuable herb that can help you transition from summer to autumn by strengthening the cardiovascular system as a whole. The best way to use hawthorn is to pick the berries, flowers and leaves dry them and make a tea. You can also purchase it in capsules.
- Tulsi (or holy basil) – works with ingredients like oats to help us 'rest and digest'.
- Coriander – fights infection and helps skin and digestive health.
- Cinnamon – is anti-inflammatory, antifungal and helps balance blood sugar.
- Ginger – aids digestion by reducing bloating, internal wind and is warming for the body.
- Chilli – supports the immune system.
- Basil – is packed with antioxidants, vitamins A and C for reducing free radicals in the body.
- Mint – good for mental health and mental fatigue.
- Marjoram – great for digestion and reducing inflammation.
- Lemon balm – a soothing herb for anxiety, digestion and the skin; it was said to be used in spells for love.
- Horseradish – is packed with minerals and vitamins, therefore helps respiratory and digestive systems and decreases inflammation in the body.
- Rosemary – is responsible for adding to our vitality with its iron content that helps to transport oxygen through the mind for clear focus and memory.
- Thyme – helps with coughs.

Herbal teas in the autumn are so rewarding as the warmth of summer subsides. See the recipes below for some ideas and why they are good for you.

French apple, honey and cinnamon tea

The combination of the sweetness of apples and the warming effect of cinnamon and honey makes this a nourishing and healing combination. Drink the tea daily at this time of year to ward off coughs and colds.

A daily dose of two or three cups is made as follows:

Ingredients

4 apples washed and sliced

2 tbsp. honey (local if possible or manuka)

1 tsp. cinnamon

Method

Cook the sliced apples in half a litre of water until they are soft – likely around 5 to 10 minutes – and strain everything into a jug. Combine the water with honey and cinnamon.

Lemon balm, rosemary and thyme tea

This tea soothes the throat and helps clear the lungs of phlegm which can cause a cough. It magically lifts the mood and restores vitality. What's not to like? I make this tea in a glass teapot or a cafetière and cover with a tea cosy to keep warm. Add a teaspoon of manuka or local honey to taste if you like after combining the ingredients below with half a litre of almost boiling water.

Ingredients

1/3 cup lemon balm, dried or fresh (soothing for anxiety)

1/3 cup rosemary (good for clarity and focus)

1 tbsp. thyme (helpful for clearing coughs)

Alicky's Magic Wand
Exercises

Bending down with knees bent swing arms gently back as far as they will go. Feel the stretch. On a deep inhale come back to standing. Swing your arms strongly upward and over your head keeping the arms straight. Again feel the stretch. Pump the hands backwards three times holding the breath then towards each other on a tiny sharp in breath three times. Swing arms back down and behind on the long out breath. Repeat as many times as you want. It gets easier with daily practice.

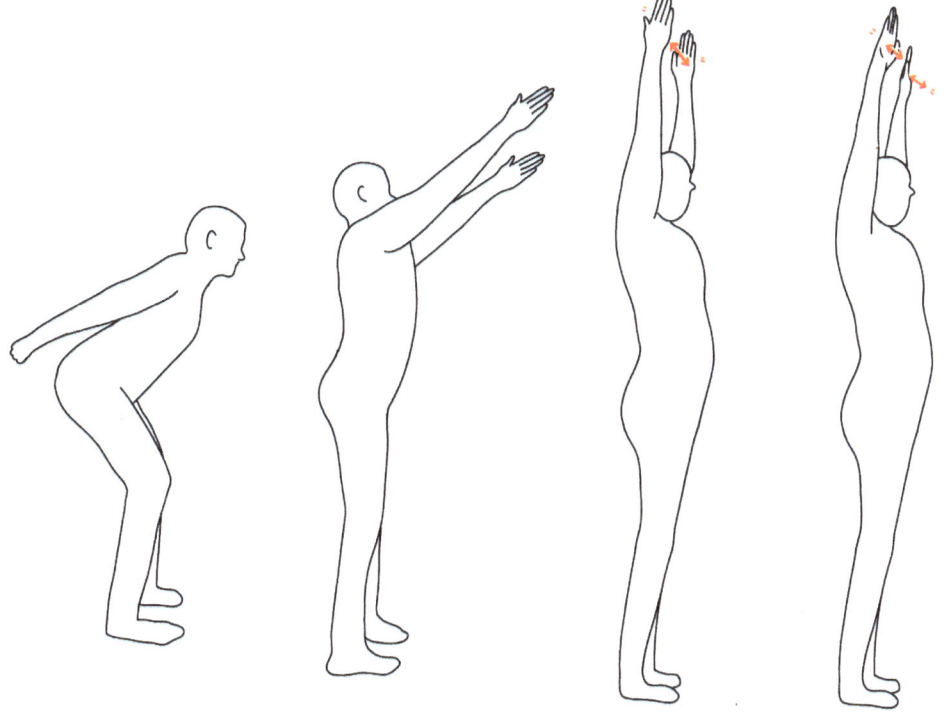

Breathe and stretch: this image shows a lung opening exercise for a quick energy boost.

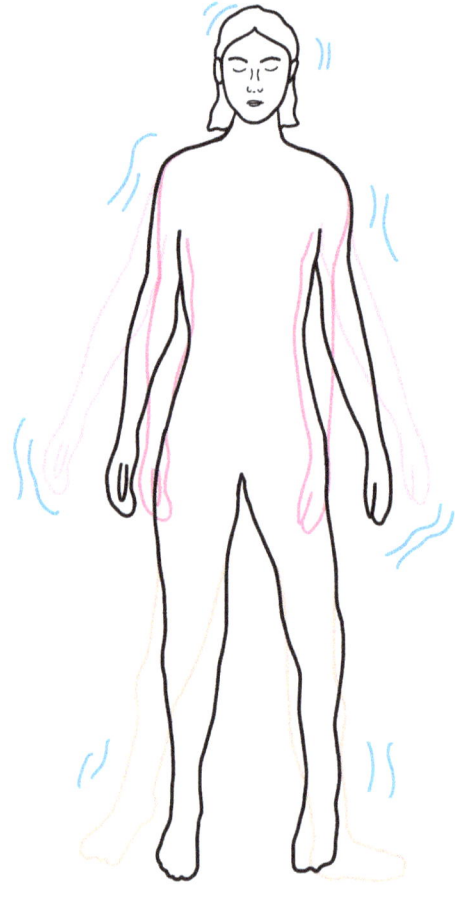

Chi gung shaking

Chi gung shaking is another brilliant exercise for getting rid of excess autumn energy. Imagine you are standing under a cold shower and shaking off all the cold water from head to toe. Emulate this activity for a few minutes and imagine shaking off the excess chi.

Moons

Late September gifts us with the harvest Moon. This powerful Moon energy leads us into autumn. It is a time to stay connected to the Earth's elements and also to remember the power of this transitional period. The Moon's energy rises to your head and can create emotional chaos energetically: depression, low mood, sadness and body exhaustion. The hunter's Moon in October glows bright for hunters to see their prey at night.

Dopamine

It is important to build up our dopamine levels during autumn as the light starts to fade. We can do this with nutrition by following the recommendations in this chapter. Dopamine is a neurotransmitter (a chemical messenger) made in your brain which enhances motivation, attention, memory and mood, including feelings of pleasure and satisfaction. An imbalance of dopamine can result in conditions such as restless leg syndrome. A complex condition like ADHD can be affected by dopamine levels dropping.

Abdominal breathing technique

Also known as hara breathing, this technique uses autumn's crisp, clear air to invigorate your body. Inhale with awareness, focusing the mind on the breath moving in and moving out. Allow your belly to expand on the in breath and relax on the out breath. You can also do this at night, which will deeply relax you and allow your intestines to relax ensuring a good evacuation in the morning! Hold your hands on the abdomen below the naval. On every breath in, push out the abdomen. Hold and release, counting to four at each breath in and hold and out.

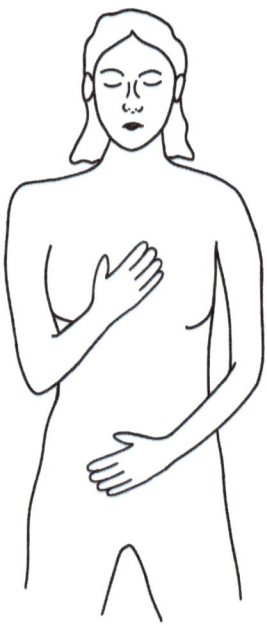

This image shows the abdominal breathing technique.

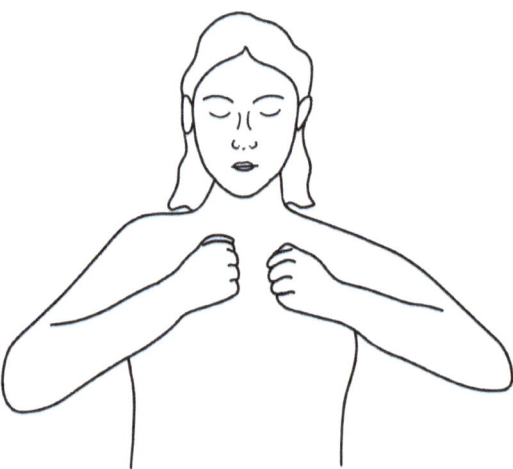

This image show how to gorilla thump your chest to energise and clear the lungs of stagnant chi.

Box breathing

Breathe in for four counts, hold for four, breathe out for four and hold for four. Box breathing is fabulous for tackling anxiety, worry, low mood and fear. You can incorporate this with the abdominal breathing by counting in and out for four if that feels good.

Gorilla thumping

With two fists, thump on your chest either side of the sternum as hard as you feel is comfortable. Meanwhile breathe in and out deeply. Thumping your chest can also stimulate the thymus, which may support the immune system and lung energy meridian.

Foot bathing

Make a mustard and ginger, or a eucalyptus and pine foot bath. Fill a washing-up bucket with hot water. Take a muslin bag (tie top with string!) and fill with chopped ginger, mustard powder (it can stain yellow) and pine needles for the full natural experience. If you don't have the natural ingredients use essential oils instead.

Self-esteem

Remember to respect yourself and others. In eastern wisdom, the lungs are linked to self-esteem, self-worth and respect for ourselves and others. Take some time to consider where you want to use your time and energy.

Declutter the mind

Having a clear out to start the season of autumn is wonderful. Let's let go of some things that don't serve us well, particularly people in our lives. Look at who supports you emotionally or drains you of energy. We change as we grow older and it is okay to observe and shift freindships. Make a list, observe it, have an opinion, then destroy it where appropriate.

Thank you

Remember to take a moment to be thankful for all you have achieved and enjoyed so far this year, no matter how big or small. Remember to thank people who have helped you along the way, negatively or positively – there is always a lesson in there!

Purpose

Pick something that gives you purpose in life. Something that energises you and excites you daily and carry this on to enhance the months ahead.

MANTRA

At the beginning of the day on waking and at the end of the day before sleep repeat: 'Thank you.'

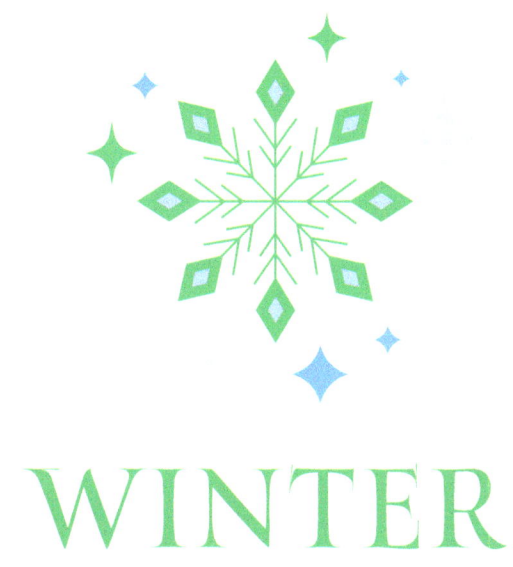

WINTER

*'Take rest. A field that has rested
gives a beautiful crop.'*
Ovid

The Season of Winter

Months: December, January, February
Winter element: Water
Organs: Kidneys and Bladder
Kidneys and Bladder active time of day: 3 p.m. to 7 p.m.

Winter is nature's way to pause, renew itself, and gather momentum for the new cycle of life. During the winter months, energy moves inwards. In the West, we tend to dread the darker nights and cold weather. But it is a great time if we can get our heads around it! Let's change that feeling of we just must 'get through it'. Look at the wonder of winter and the gifts it brings. How can we align with it? There can be simple joy in knowing that the darkness will end and the light will return as it always does!

This season is connected energetically to the water element in Chinese wisdom. The organs to look after are the kidney and bladder. Our kidney energy particularly houses our wisdom and vital energy. I call it the power bank. It likes to stay warm and be nourished.

Winter is a time of contracting energy (conserving energy for the year ahead). It is a time for slowing down, reflection, meditation and writing, chi gung, yoga and walking.

On the 21st of December the winter solstice arrives in the northern hemisphere with the shortest day and the longest night of the year. After the solstice, from the 22nd December, energy starts rising and expanding again. You hear people saying,

'Thank heavens, the days will start getting longer!' The further south you go, clearly, this is not the case since the equator has equal hours of day and night. I lived on the equator for a few years and certainly missed the change in daylight hours!

The Boons and Banes of Winter

This chart gives a brief outline of the ups and downs of your emotions in wintertime. An interesting way to check in and see how you're feeling now.

BOONS	BANES
Enjoying warmth: cozying up, fires, earlier bedtimes	Hibernation time: everything feels like it's come to a halt
Time for reflection	Less daylight and dopamine bringing sadness and low mood
Emotional nourishment from warm foods	Increased appetite if feeling undernourished emotionally
Addressing fears and phobias	Fearful
Good time for knowledge and gaining wisdom	Low motivation and energy for life

The Physical During Winter

Organs involved in winter: kidneys and bladder

Active times of the organ

Kidneys: 5 p.m. to 7 p.m.

Bladder: 1 p.m. to 3 p.m.

During winter, the physical aspect of our health is linked to the kidneys and bladder. They both play a vital role in maintaining our body's balance.

The kidneys especially have a busy role keeping us healthy and helping us age well. Our kidneys act as a filtration system, removing waste products from the blood through urine and sweat. They maintain body fluid at the correct levels of safety for the body to function. They regulate the body's salt, potassium and acid content, and cleverly release hormones that regulate our blood pressure. Vitamin D production by the kidneys vitally promotes strong healthy bones.

In eastern understanding the kidneys house the vital energy of the mind, body and soul. The power bank! Also they house our unique wisdom and the emotion of fear.

Our bladder literally holds our urine ready for peeing. It is a muscular organ and acts as a balloon. It can hold approximately 200–300 ml of urine. In eastern understanding the bladder also holds fear, like the kidneys.

Physical imbalance of the kidneys may lead to:

- Thirsty, dry mouth
- Dark-coloured urine
- Dry stools, constipation
- Night sweats and nightmares
- Thinning hair
- Vertigo and dizziness

Balanced kidneys lead to these physical benefits:

- A strong sense of knowing
- Positive mental strength
- Strong willpower
- Ambitious character
- Clear lightly coloured urine (like white wine!)

Physical imbalance of the bladder may lead to:

- Dark and excessive urine
- Lower back pain
- Indication of kidney issues

A balanced bladder leads to these physical benefits:

- Regular and clear urine
- Pain-free and strong lower back
- Strength to overcome fear

Keeping your kidney area warm in winter is really important for good health and strength at this time. Look at the table of foods to nurture you in winter to help guide you to a balanced diet through the wintertime. Be aware of your body's acidity too. You can test this with a kit or ask the doctor to test it for you. If you have kidney infections or cystitis (connected to the bladder) then keep the body alkaline. Stress will have a severe effect on the acidity of the body and can cause these infections.

The Emotional During Winter

The kidneys are the unsung heroes of the body and are yin in essence; the bladder is yang in essence. Remember, opposites create balance: yin/yang, hot/cold, contract/expand.

As our chi moves inwards, we can reflect on the deep, introspective nature of winter. This season encourages us to look at our fears, deal with them and confront the shadows within. Look at this as a time of great opportunities for knowledge and learning.

Organ time is interesting with the kidney's peak hours being from 5 p.m. to 7 p.m. and the bladder's from 1 p.m. to 3 p.m. Having some understanding of the rhythms can help in aligning our physical and emotional health.

In western and eastern wisdom, these organs are significant for our survival and are vital to nurture. The bladder, being yang in essence, is a reservoir of energy storage, a bit like your savings account. Instead of storing money it is storing your energy. So it's important to slow down and nourish, then you can flourish in winter. Act as if you were hibernating – like the trees and seeds of plants that head underground and rest. Your wisdom is held in your kidney energy. Strong kidney chi/energy equals strong willpower! This willpower is vital at the time of the new year for all those resolutions we make and seeds of ideas that we plant in our mind for the year ahead. Nurturing the energy of the kidneys provides us with wisdom and the vital energy required for daily life.

Causes of energy depletion

Tiredness in the late afternoon from 5 p.m. to 7 p.m. is a sign you are depleted in kidney chi. And the same feeling between 1 p.m. and 3 p.m. is a sign of depleted bladder chi.

Try to keep your feet and ankles warm, as well as the waistline where the kidneys and bladder are located. Fear; anxiety; shock; stress and overtiredness; nervousness; prolonged physical exhaustion; chronic illness; chronic pain; too much sexual activity; multiple pregnancies close together; excess of salt in the diet will all exhaust your energy.

These are signs that your kidney chi is low:

- Lack of willpower
- Lack of sexual desire
- Lack of motivation and zest for life
- Lack of direction
- Tiredness
- Early grey hair
- Self-doubt
- Thinning hair
- Memory loss
- Always cold

EFT to Reduce Feelings of Fear

When our kidneys are not functioning energetically well we can feel fear and low energy. Make a note of any emotions around fear or low energy and choose the most charged one, the feeling that resonates with you now. Observe the feeling or mood that is present and taking up your headspace. Notice where you feel it most in your body. How intense is it? Give the feeling a title, e.g. 'My fear of ...'

This is a quick script to release fear and should take roughly three minutes, depending on the level of feeling!

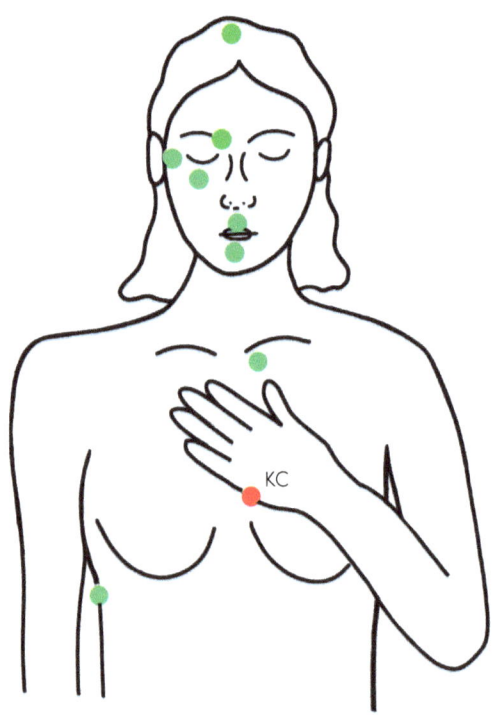

The nine points to tap when practising EFT.

1. Give the level and intensity of your fear a mark first: zero (nothing at all) to ten (extreme intensity).

2. Take three slow, deep breaths in and out before you begin.

3. Tapping on the side of the hand, on the karate-chop point, say your set-up phrase three times as below. (We only use the karate-chop point on the side of the hand to say the set-up statement.)

> *'Even though I am feeling fearful right now, I deeply and completely accept myself anyway.'*
>
> *'Even though I am feeling fearful right now, I deeply and completely accept and honour myself anyway.'*
>
> *'Even though I am feeling fearful at the moment, I deeply and completely accept myself anyway, and acknowledge I feel this fear.'*

4. Start tapping on the points around the face and body shown on the diagram above. Begin at the eyebrow point and move from point to point after each script line and say:

> *Inner eye: 'My fear feeling.'*
> *Side of eye: 'My fear feeling.'*
> *Under eye: 'I feel so frightened.'*
> *Under nose: 'I am scared.'*
> *Chin: 'I am scared about ...' (e.g. a challenge ahead or just life.)*
> *Collar bone: 'I feel so fearful.'*
> *Under arm: 'My fear feeling.'*
> *Top of head: 'I am frightened.'*

5. Now change the wording to start letting go of a feeling that's more specific in the next round of tapping: what is the fear really about? Exams? Failing?

A job interview? Tap around the points in the same order as above starting at the inner eybrow point:

'I choose to let this fear about ... go.'
'I choose to release this fear of ... from every part of me.'
'It's OK to feel fear of ... but now I choose to let it go.'
'It's OK to have this feeling of fear about ... but now I choose to release it from my ...' (wherever it may be in the body.)

Where do you feel this fear feeling now? Has it moved somewhere else in the head or body?

6. Next, start tapping again, guiding the mind to where the feeling is in your body. Keep tapping around the points in the same pattern as above, and use relevant words for where you may feel it now. It can move quickly, so follow it! For example:

'This feeling in my tummy.'
'This feeling in my head.'
'This feeling in my chest.'
'This feeling is moving to my ...'

This tapping can release tears, yawning and tiredness when we start releasing the fear and emotions and this is good news. Keep tapping until the physical and emotional feeling has cleared.

7. Now, tune into the feeling again. It may have changed to another feeling and that's also good. You can play with different words to suit your feeling in that moment. Tap on this remaining feeling using relevant words similar to these:

'My remaining fear.'
' I am now feeling ...'
'I still have this fear feeling but it's less now.'

'My remaining low energy with this fear.'
'I now feel better, lighter and clearer.'

Take three deep breaths, counting in for four and out for four.

8. Check your level of feeling again. Hopefully, the number has reduced dramatically. If there are any remaining feelings around your fear feeling, then do another round of tapping. It's OK to change the wording. As I have said before, just check the emotional and physical feelings. Then you can tap on where the feeling is now. Perhaps your 'fear feeling' is in your tummy, chest, or back, which are typical places to feel your fear. Follow the feeling if it moves around the body – it does tend to before disappearing! Do you feel clearer now? Perhaps tap in some positives for the healing to increase, such as:

'I can be brave and see through the fear.'
'I choose to let go of this bad fear feeling with my new energy coming through and the wisdom I have gained.'
'I choose to listen to my fear and notice that I can release it easily at this time.'

Fear can be very heavy and old so try observing how you feel the following day having done this tapping session. Perhaps you notice you are feeling happier, lighter, less burdened. This is wonderful and the magic of the energy psychology work of EFT!

This completes the session.

Food to Nurture you in Winter

The winter months are generally colder with fewer daylight hours. Cold food can be damaging for our kidney and bladder energy. The natural energy at this time of year is inward, therefore keep the warmth inside you. So focus on hot food, whole grains and hot drinks. You may find your food intake increases and that is OK.

FOOD TO INCLUDE
Bone or vegetable broth
Chicken
Ginger and cardamom
Rice
Aduki and black beans
Root vegetables
Celery
Pumpkin seeds
Sunflower seeds
Vitamins C and D and Zinc
Goji berries, blueberries, blackberries (makes a great whisky infusion), mulberries, elderberries
Grapes and raisins
Dark-skinned fruit, including the list above, also beetroot and dark chocolate
Probiotics

WINTER

RECIPES FOR WINTER

Gomasio salt

Gomasio salt is a staple in the East. This recipe is brilliant to use in place of pure salt at your table. It is also a very popular gift!

Ingredients

1 part sea salt (please use good-quality flaky sea salt as it adds texture)
1 part nori seaweed flakes (helps eliminate toxins)
20 parts white or black sesame seeds (liver and kidney protection, high in anti-inflammatory and antioxidant nutrients)

Method

Toast the sesame seeds until golden brown but watch them carefully to avoid burning, add the seaweed flakes and warm through.

Leave to cool before grinding them in a pestle and mortar or small mixer.

Mix in the salt.

Ultimate healing chicken soup

Serves 4 to 6

My ultimate chicken soup never ceases to surprise me in how effective it is at boosting your chi. It makes people feel more alive, motivated and energised! The broth that comes from cooking chicken bones boosts immunity, promotes gut repair and helps the digestive system to better absorb nutrients. If you don't want chicken, you can try using tofu or experiment with other plant-based alternatives. I tend to freeze any excess soup for another day, so it's always ready for emergencies!

The spring onion, garlic, and ginger all help warm the body and energise your digestive system. Ginger helps with nausea and indigestion too! Turmeric is anti-inflammatory. Adding root vegetables in with the chicken will support and stabilise blood sugar and your energy, reducing pesky sweet cravings. I add other seasonal veggies through the year. For example, in summer I add peas and sweetcorn that taste sweet so help cravings and also support and balance blood sugars. In autumn, add rice, making it almost like a congee, which is extremely healing for the large intestine and lungs. In winter, I add barley, aduki or black beans to boost the kidney energy.

Ingredients

1 tbsp. extra virgin olive oil
4 spring onions, thinly sliced (high mineral content)
1 head of garlic, peeled and sliced (a great all-round healer)
5-cm piece of ginger, peeled and grated (warming and energising)
2.5-cm piece of turmeric, peeled and sliced into thin rounds (anti-inflammatory)
3 stalks celery sliced thinly on a bias (calming and packed with vitamin C)
2 carrots, sliced (improves vision, balances blood sugar, boosts immunity and brain health)

13-cm piece of lemongrass, bruised by smashing with the butt of a kitchen knife (helps sore throats and allergies)

2 sprigs fresh rosemary (disinfectant for the mouth)

3 sprigs fresh thyme (helps soothe coughs)

3 tbsp. fresh oregano leaves chopped or 1 tbsp. of dried oregano (soothes bronchitis)

3 litres (or less, if you prefer a thicker soup) of water or stock (chicken or vegetable)

450g organic chicken stripped or in pieces (great source of protein)

2 tsp. black pepper (helps absorption of nutrients)

1 star anise pod (helps to calm the nerves and to help with flatulence)

Method

In a very large stockpot or soup pan, heat the oil over medium to high heat. Add the onions, garlic and ginger, and allow to sweat for 3 minutes or until translucent.

Add the turmeric, celery, carrots, lemongrass and the herbs and cook for 2 minutes.

Stir in the chicken strips or pieces, then add water or stock. Bring to boil and simmer for one hour. When the soup is ready, remove the lemongrass and star anise plus any hard stems as its not nice to chew on them!

Season with soy sauce. Sometimes I add miso, especially in the winter to support the kidney energy.

Immune booster juice

These are ginger and lemon shots, so serve in small glasses.

Ingredients

One small apple (aids digestion)
Lemon with pith (alkalising)
A small chunk of ginger, adjust the dose as to how brave you are feeling! (Ginger is commonly used to stimulate circulation and get the blood moving throughout the body to prevent stagnation.)

Method

Juice the ingredients in a juicer and pour into the shot glasses. I would drink up in one gulp! For an anti-inflammatory boost, add turmeric chopped fresh or as a powder or tincture.

You can freeze this juice in ice-cube trays, so they are handy when needed.

Hot toddy

Alcohol can be beneficial in small doses when we are ill and can actually shift energy and dampness through the body.

Dissolve honey in hot water in a small pan over a low heat. Cool a little and add the immune booster juice from the recipe before plus a few leaves of sage. Finish with a small dash of whisky.

Herbs

Making warm, simple teas in the winter months will nourish us and also support our immune system with their individual healing properties. So I recommend the following recipes for helping us through the winter.

Mood-lifting tea

The spice in this tea dispels cold and depression too, bringing back vitality and inducing a calm state of mind. This is especially important during the long, dark winter evenings.

Ingredients

2 cups water
4 black peppercorns (stimulating)
4 cardamom pods (cardamom lifts your energy up to warm and restore you)
1 cinnamon stick (balances blood sugar and is anti-inflammatory)
4 cloves (calming and antiviral)
A few slices of root ginger (warming)
Milk and/or honey to taste

Method

Place water and spices into a pan and bring to a near boil. Cover and simmer for an hour. Strain and serve. Enjoy two or three cups daily.

Sore throat tea

The common cold can be a nuisance in winter. Sage is excellent for sore throats, especially tonsilitis; it has vitamin C in high doses and vitamin D. You could add oat straw, hawthorn, rosemary or coriander to this tea.

Ingredients

4–5 sage leaves (also protect against neurodegenerative disease and cognitive dysfunction)
½ squeezed lemon (alkalising)
A teaspoon of local or manuka honey (good all-rounder!)
Vitamin C powder (good immune booster)
Vitamin D drops (good immune booster)

Method

Put all the ingredients into a teapot or cafetiere and pour over hot, not boiling, water. Leave to steep for at least 4 minutes. This tea can be drunk warm or sipped when cooled through the day.

WINTER

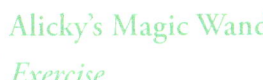 Alicky's Magic Wand
Exercise

Quieter, more mindful exercise is needed in winter to bring the energy inwards, for example, yin yoga, chi gung, or mindful walking. Swimming in fresh water or even just being near water can immediately help boost your kidney energy. And make sure to get outside and moving when the Sun is up! Try a gentle meditation exercise like the one below.

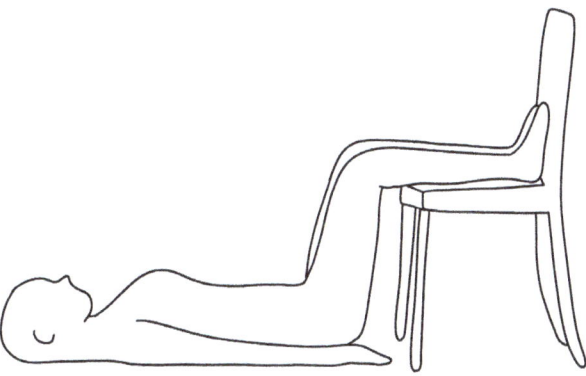

This image shows a great lying down position for rebooting your energy.

Resting or lying down meditation

The kidney meridian runs through the back of the legs: from the soles of the feet up to the kidneys in the lower back. So, getting into a position lying down with your feet up at a ninety-degree angle allows the energy to flow from the feet back into the kidneys. This gives the kidneys a boost of energy. Stay in this position for a minimum of twenty minutes. Listen to a meditation script or just breathe mindfully and slowly. Also, try the box breathing in the autumn chapter page 85.

Moons

The cold Moon appears in December near the time of winter solstice in the northern hemisphere. Use this time for a moment of introspection and reflection. Always remember the full Moon energy is powerful in different ways throughout each season. This is an opportunity to tune in to how you really feel and know that this is what may need releasing. EFT tapping is a great way of shifting emotions and energy that may be heavy at this time.

Light therapy

Getting sunlight where possible to raise dopamine levels is crucial! Consider using light-therapy glasses or a lamp for artificial sunlight if you feel you need some perking up in the dark wintery days or if you often suffer from SAD. I love my light-therapy glasses and put them on first thing in the morning and wear them whilst making my coffee, feeding my dogs, ironing, tidying or reading.

Keep warm

Keep your lower back and feet warm. A hot-water bottle is great for warming the lower back – you can slip it behind you while sitting at your desk. Invest in some good socks; wear a thick scarf and hat if it's cold outside. Drink ginger tea, enjoy warm soups, have a hot bath or sauna when you can!

Foot bathing

A foot bath with grated ginger in the water is an excellent way of boosting kidney energy. Use a washing-up bowl and add grated or chopped ginger or ginger essential oil to the water. Sit for twenty minutes with your feet soaking in the water. You can add other essential oils and give yourself a foot scrub and moisturise afterwards.

Sleep

Have a hot bath before bed, maybe try a hot-water bottle at your feet when sleeping.

Aim for a 10 p.m. bedtime. If you get tired in the day, try a short meditation nap for half an hour, especially between 5 p.m. and 7 p.m. for an energy boost. This will be nurturing for your kidney energy, which don't forget is your power bank!

Wisdom

Listen to inspirational talks – they can increase your wisdom! Face your fears with EFT to help you recognise your negative emotions and replace them with a positive outcome.

Moonstone

This is the crystal of new beginnings; it is great for wintertime. The moonstone symbolises balance and harmony and helps you connect to your intuition and power.

MANTRA

'I only accept what is good for my higher self and take back my power today.'

Now For a Bit of Fun!

Now, take a moment to look at how you are nourishing yourself and cultivating your wisdom throughout each year. See if you can answer these questions:

Which is your favourite season overall?

How do you know this is the best season for you?

We can observe the world through our five senses: seeing, feeling, hearing, smelling and tasting. Being aware of your senses will significantly improve your communication with the world around you. This section of the book is about the body and how it can never lie. Have some fun with this information. Body shapes, hands, handwriting and our faces all give us away. Our tone of voice, our eye movements and smell – they all tell a tale! Have a go at exploring this a little and see how you get on!

Facial diagnosis (Book Michio Kushi)

The basic concept of face reading is an ancient Chinese practice that looks at the face to assess emotional and physical health. This technique dates back 4,000 years. Practitioners of Chinese medicine will use the information gained from a facial reading as a guide to aiding your health.

It is believed that areas of the face can indicate problems with certain organs. Face reading looks at everything on the outside as a direct indication of emotional issues and physical ailments.

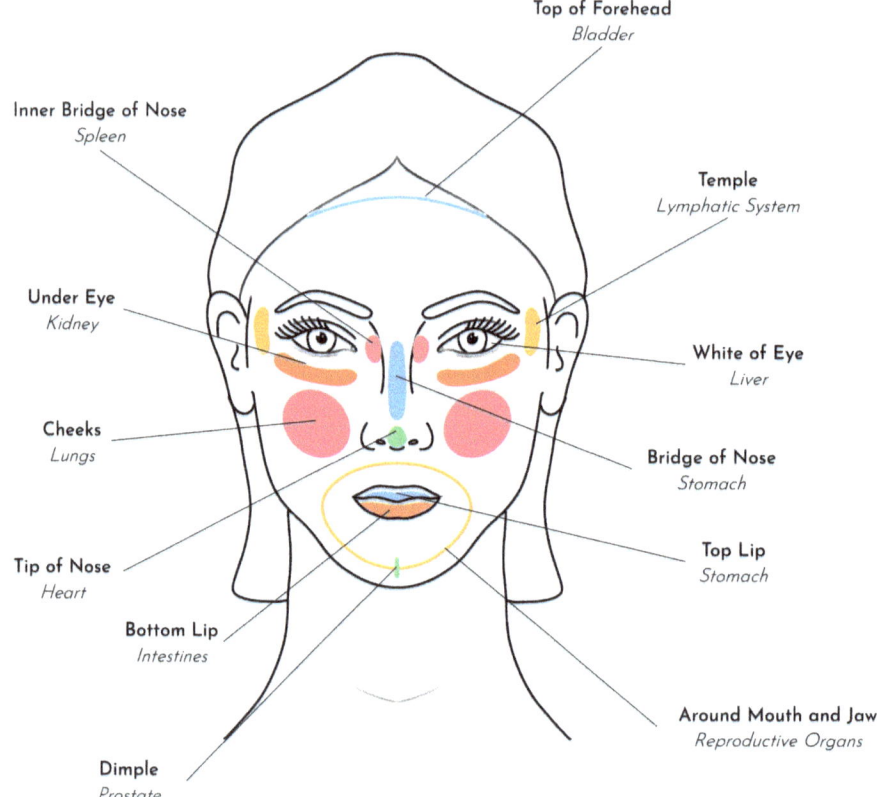

Map of the facial areas for diagnosis.

The left side of the face shows the real personality while the right side shows the person we present to the world. A symmetrical face reveals a balanced personality.

If your left side is lifted and clear-looking this shows the real personality.

If your right side looks tighter and more scrutinous this shows a distrust for your surroundings possibly through your experience in life.

The opposite can be also true. If your right side is glowing and clear, this is the side you show out to the world.

If your left side is tired-looking and tighter; this is the real internal person.

Obviously, in simple western terms, we can see from someone's facial expression whether they are sad or happy, grumpy or away with the fairies. Let's dive in for some fun!

Eyes

The eyes talk and tell us a lot about the liver and about your spirit and connection to life. Is there vibrancy or deadness in your eyes? Their shape will dictate a lot of characteristics. Large and round eyes indicate cheerfulness and joy. Small eyes show more control, perhaps the person is careful. Deep-set eyes show the person is good at dealing with issues but won't necessarily share their feelings. Eyes that turn up at the edge show a positive personality. Eyes that turn down show sadness and indicate the person is private.

Red veins or a yellowing in the whites of the eyes suggests a stagnation and inflammation of the liver and possibly other organs.

Darkness at the inner eye socket is a sign of weak spleen energy. This can indicate a lack of emotional and physical nurturing as a child.

Dark circles under the eyes indicate the kidneys are struggling and need some TLC. Puffy bags indicate excess liquid or mucus in the system. Kidney energy does weaken as we age, so it is even more vital to look after our kidneys as we get older. Check out the winter season chapter for more on the kidneys.

Eyebrows

Shorter eyebrows indicate an inability to digest fats; thinner or soft brows suggest liver stress. Eyebrows that don't grow wide across the face, i.e. there is a missing area at the end, indicate thyroid issues.

Ladder lines and redness between the eyebrows indicate agitation or stagnation in the liver. One line indicates a personal crisis may have occurred – this will impact your health so watch out. Two lines are OK but indicate there may be bouts of anger that flash out.

Three lines tell us you need to be careful! You may be too focused on achieving a goal and over consume alcohol and fats; you need to look after yourself.

The corners of the forehead, by the temples, represent bladder issues. Grooves, lines and growths of progressive acne in this area are an indication of an imbalance in your bladder chi.

Nose

The heart is represented by the nose. The tip of the nose is a prominent marker of heart health. Red visible veins and excess sweat are all signs of imbalance in the heart. Perhaps some hypertension is present. A pockmarked nose indicates too much alcohol consumption. It also indicates your relationship with money. Wide nose wings can show someone who handles money well. The wider the nose the bigger the heart is, emotionally. A downturned nose suggests someone who is business focused and entrepreneurial. An upturned nose signifies a playful person who is a good listener.

Cheeks

The cheeks can represent the lungs generally. Clear skin here indicates good health. Flushed cheeks may indicate excess liquid, sugar and drugs. A greyness will indicate grief and possibly a liver disorder. Brown marks on the skin show too much sugar consumption. Cheek dimples are considered cute, and people who have them tend get away with murder!! Pimples on the cheeks will tell you that there is too much fat and dairy in your diet.

Mouth

Your mouth should ideally be the same width as your nose.

Your lips represent different parts of your digestive system. The upper lip reflects the condition of the stomach and spleen. It should be moist, pink, slightly red. This indicates good health. Pale lips will show low chi.

The lower lip is about the intestine. Irritated skin in the corners of the mouth like cold sores is about the duodenum (first section of the small intestine) and can indicate diarrhoea and loose stools.

Thin lips can indicate an excess of meat has been eaten. Swollen lips can indicate a weak spleen energy.

Tightness in the mouth indicates a tight intestine and tight vagina too. Women may have issues giving birth. A large wide mouth may indicate a woman who will give birth easily!

Dryness or chapped lips will be signs of constipation and intestinal dysfunction.

Skin

Lung issues will show up on skin that may be dry, cheeks may be sallow or very pale, pockmarked with open pores. Clear, unblemished cheeks indicate good health, especially good lung energy.

Wrinkles

These indicate a weakness in the energy of the heart and small intestine. This is due to a slow circulation in the heart.

Dimples

A dimple on the chin can show you are lucky.

Jaw

A strong jaw shows a person is intuitive, spontaneous and sometimes impulsive! Also strong and courageous, with a tendency to be stubborn. Sagging jawlines also indicate weakness in the kidney energy.

Chin

Deep horizontal creases between the lips and the chin indicate you are burning out – slow down. Hairy chins on women are hormonal and indicate too many fats are being ingested.

The Hands

Your hands represent your strengths and weaknesses.

Large, square palms indicate you are a yang person: you are strong and resilient with strong muscles and you like action, therefore, you will want to eat more protein, especially meat.

Slimmer palms indicate a more yin person: quieter in nature and less active naturally, with less muscle bulk. This indicates that a more plant-based diet would suit you.

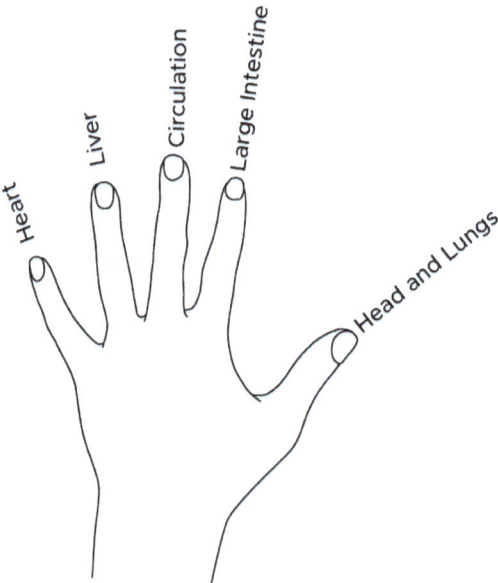

This image shows which fingers are linked to which organ in the body.

Short, thicker fingers also indicate a yang constitution: strong, outspoken, and possibly quite loud. Thinner, elongated fingers indicate a quieter more sensitive personality, more prone to be artistic and creative in nature.

Your thumb represents your head and lungs energy. Any white bumps here indicate too much dairy in the system. If there are red bumps, especially in the muscle below the thumb the person consumes too much sugar and spicy foods. If the person is depressed, then palpate the point in the centre of the thumb pad and pull hard or hold tightly and breathe.

The index finger represents the large intestine. Squeezing hard and palpating the point between the base of the thumb and index finger helps the intestines evacuate. This action also relieves headaches.

The middle finger represents the circulatory functions but also can send energy to your sex organs. Rotating the finger and massaging it can help. It can also be used to overcome vertigo in an emergency – bend the finger backwards and breathe deeply.

The ring finger represents the liver and gall bladder, so when you feel you have toxic elements in your system massage the finger all over and rotate it to get energy there and increase blood circulation.

The little finger represents the heart and small intestine. If the tip of the little finger is red, then there is too much energy in the heart. If there is numbness, then please get your heart checked by a doctor. In ancient times, if a person experienced a heart attack or stroke, they were told to bite the end of their little finger to restart the heart energy. This was a long time before defibrillators, clearly! I would probably use this as first aid if a person fainted.

Handwriting

Have a go at some free writing in a journal. Try to write how you would naturally. Come back to your writing in about half an hour and observe the details and shapes of the words you wrote. Are they slanting forwards or backwards? Are they round or jagged? The size of a person's handwriting is key. I would guess that large expansive letters indicate that you are yang in nature and smaller spindly writing suggests you are yin. In addition, the size of handwriting can show the writer's need for attention. Large handwriting suggests extroversion, a desire to be noticed. Small handwriting suggests introversion and attention to detail.

The slant of the handwriting is often associated with emotional expression. Right-slanted writing indicates a passionate, confident and outgoing personality. Left-slanted writing may show introspection and reserved emotions, possibly a slightly depressed character.

When you receive a letter, you will unconsciously be feeling what that person is all about just through interpreting their handwriting. Large, round, circular writing perhaps shows an open and generous person who wears their heart on their sleeve. Small, spiky, spider script might indicate a more internal-focused person not prone to sharing feelings and perhaps they are living in their head – being logical and practical. Let's bring back letter writing!

The writing of a person can also tell you about their yin and yang. A yang person will have strong, large writing, enjoy writing with a bold felt tip pen or fountain pen; they may write in capitals. A yin-type person will prefer lighter, smaller more curly writing using a pencil or thin-tipped pen.

Have fun diagnosing your friends through their letter or card writing. See how correct you are!

Body Shapes

Observations about body shapes are fascinating. Let's start by looking at the standard ratio of the head to the body that is 1:7. If the head appears small then the constitution of that person will be weak. If the head seems large then the constitution will be strong.

Taller people tend to be more yin in personality, quiet and thoughtful, while and smaller people are more yang, loud and less perceptive.

Also, we can look at the five elements theory of the body, connecting organs to the elements of fire, water, earth, metal and wood. Certain body characteristics indicate a link to the energy and function of certain organs.

Kidney and bladder energy: Water element

Body shape: weaker lower back and buttocks, a little saggy.
Qualities: more likely to be artistic and creative, a dreamer; easy personality; works better alone.
Downfalls: fearful, can be timid; a worrier, gets drained around too many people for a long period of time; often late; lacks motivation; prone to fear of failure and self-doubt. In extreme cases they may have night sweats.

Lungs and large intestine: Metal element

Body shape: small shoulders, small abdomen. May have excess body hair.

Qualities: Full of vitality, cool-headed, intuitive. Easily adjusts to different environments. Stands straight and may have a loud voice.

Downfalls: holds sadness; can have hunched shoulders as if carrying all the world's problems. Weak voice. Risk avoidant.

Heart and small intestine: Fire element

Body shape: heart-shaped face, smaller hands and feet.

Qualities: loyal, predictable, and unconditionally loving.

Downfalls: easily taken advantage of; easily unsettled; can suffer from heart palpitations.

Stomach and spleen: Earth element

Body shape: pear-shaped, rounded buttocks.

Qualities: secure, loyal, faithful; sense of responsibility.

Downfalls: worries too much; can suffer from tummy aches; self-sacrificing.

Liver and gall bladder: Wood element

Body shape: broad, squared shoulders, slender body, straight back and defined facial features.

Qualities: self-reliant, resilient; intelligent and stable. A list-maker who likes to be organised.

Downfalls: disorganised; tendency to be an irritable person. Possibility of being a control freak, 'it's my way or the highway' attitude.

Dreams

Dreams may be the seeds of our future vision, our ideas about who we are and what we want. Dreaming about the life we want crystallises our vision and helps us to find ways to materialise all we need, to have another go at doing our best over the coming year.

I am no dream expert so won't go into depth here, but it is important to stay in tune with the connection between organs and emotions, as listed in the body types section above. Often we have frightening dreams if our kidneys or bladder need attention, because these organs hold one's fear. The liver and gall bladder hold one's anger; the stomach and spleen represent nurture; lungs and large intestine, our sadness; and the heart and small intestine hold our love.

DREAM	ORGANS INVOLVED
Frightening	Kidney and bladder
Angry	Liver and gall bladder
In need of nurturing	Stomach and spleen
Sadness and death	Lung and large intestine
Love	Heart and small intestine

Conclusion

My wish for you, the reader, is that you can draw some wisdom from my writings by honouring the seasons and cycles in your life, connecting to nature and the energy it provides.

This book provides a bridge between western and eastern life principles, drawing from both to bring a unique way of living happily and healthily through the seasonal year.

I have included a brief overview of how we look at the body and mind in both cultures. This is a guide to nourish ourselves with ancient and modern wisdom. With some wisdom, we can begin to understand energy, how it is relevant to our body and mind, and the impact on the way we live. I have suggested different techniques to integrate the mind and body to stay in balance and harmony throughout the seasons. I hope this will encourage you to explore more avenues of health and healing for yourself and be open to possibilities as we just keep learning every day.

I have given you lots of fun and easy ideas and daily energy techniques to keep you in tip-top condition during the ever-changing seasons. These exercises and techniques should be practised regularly so they become normal for you wherever you are, especially if you are travelling, as this is often when you most need them at your fingertips.

I hope you notice this book winking at you from a table or bookshelf somewhere and have a quick flick through the relevant season for a healthier, happier outcome. Have fun with this exploration: smile and be happy. Go forth, be brave and try it out. Strive to be more connected to yourself and the seasonal rhythms of life.

My gift to you is hope. Hope that you will learn something from this book.

Hope that you will smile and see the simplicity in this book when living with the seasons naturally.

Hope that you will live a happy and more balanced life in each season after reading this book.

He who has health has hope; he who has hope has everything.'
ARABIAN PROVERB

Last word ...

I'm not sure who said this, but I find it very useful when thinking about my life through the seasons:

'Living a perfect life imperfectly should not be a journey to the grave with the intention of arriving looking attractive, but rather to skid sideways in with a glass of something in hand saying "WOOHOO what a ride that was!"'

Additional Resources

Brindle, Katie, *Yang Sheng: The Art of Chinese Self-Healing* (London, 2019).

Stuart-Smith, Sue, *The Well-Gardened Mind* (London, 2020) for gardening and mental health.

Hamilton, David, *I Heart Me: The Science of Self-Love* (London, 2015).

Hamilton, David, *The Five Side Effects of Kindness: The science of kindness and its impact on us.* (London, 2017).

Leendertz, Lia, *The Almanac: A seasonal guide to 2025* (London, 2024).

Hulin, Joey, *Your Spiritual Almanac: A Year of Living Mindfully* (London, 2021).

Gallagher, Kirsty, *Sacred Seasons: Nature-inspired rituals, wisdom and self-care for every day of the year* (London, 2023).

Ni, Maoshing (trans.), *The Yellow Emperor's Classic of Medicine* (Boston MA, 1995). A book on health and disease, said to have been written by the famous Chinese emperor Huang Di in around 2600 BC.

Connelly, Dianne, *Traditional Acupuncture: The Law of Five Elements* (1979).

McIntyre, Anne, *Healing Drinks* (London, 2000).

Kushi, Michio, *Your Body Never Lies: The complete book of orient diagnosis* (New York, 2007).

Acknowledgements

I am extremely grateful to Whitefox for trusting in my first project and Sarah Rouse for guiding me to the finishing line with such patience and grace.

My heartfelt thanks to the team involved: Karen Lilje for her magical typesetting, Heike Schüssler for creating the beautiful the cover design to attract my readers like a moth(!), Louise Tucker for her beady eyed copy-editing and Jill Sawyer for proofreading the book to make sure it was ready for print.

I would like to mention and send special love to my family for listening to the ranting and supporting me through the choppy waters of creating a book!

Thanks to Mali Gravell for offering her time with her constant guidance and hand holding when I struggled with technology, content and images!

To my friends who have remained interested in this project and kept me going. You know who you are.

Lastly, to Nicky, who gave me the confidence to be brave and rebrand myself, to get out there and remember who I am. An expert. I miss your wisdom and faith deeply.

About the Author

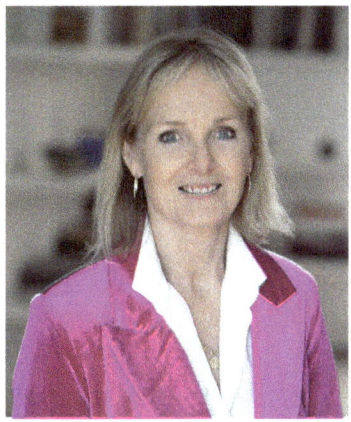

Alicky was always searching for something. She was never quite satisfied with only what was in front of her, but she was intrigued by cultures that followed a way of living that seemed an improvement on the western way of life. Alicky finds people fascinating and looks at how they choose to live or adapt to their current circumstances. People are supremely clever and yet supremely daft and destructive at the same time! This curiosity led to furthering her education, leading her to share and inspire.

Alicky's further education came after living and working in Africa where she became very unwell. Western medicine failed her. In fact, it made her condition worse at the time. She then met a truly wonderful healer through a friend who gifted her a healing session for her birthday. The results from this treatment inspired her to enrol in a three-year diploma in Traditional Chinese Medicine and shiatsu. This new beginning completely changed the course of her life.

Over the next several years, Alicky trained in nutrition, reflexology, Emotional Freedom Technique, NLP, hypnosis, InterX neurostimulation and bioenergetic healing. The gut and mental health have been at the forefront of Alicky's therapy since reading a book called *The Gut and Psychology Syndrome*

(GAP) by Dr Natasha Campbell-McBride. This was a long time before the link between the gut and mental health become widely talked about and perhaps accepted. She combines all aspects of healing the physical body with InterX and infrared therapy.

Alicky has become known as an integrated mind and body therapist. She is dedicated to helping others find their way through ill health as well as mental and physical pain in her clinic. She is also a keynote speaker for corporate wellness programmes and events, including wellness talks and retreats. Alicky's aim is to educate others in a simple and passionate way.

The journey of her interests and learning is ongoing.

www.ingramcontent.com/pod-product-compliance
Lightning Source LLC
Chambersburg PA
CBHW061149070526
44584CB00034B/4465